Advanced Praise

Even though I've never had a broken neck, I was surprised to find that I was able to relate to some of Sarah's experiences.

—Luellen Hooper

Sarah's account of her accident and the long process of recovery is inspiring.

—Niki Lonjers

Sarah's humor and insight will make those life-altering months after an illness or injury more bearable for those in a similar predicament. An entertainingly relatable and humorous look at the recovery process.

—Jess Gould

Sarah's writing is easy to read. I feel like we're sitting down having a cup of coffee or a bowl of ice cream and you are telling me the story of your broken neck.

—Ginger Montgomery

Although it was written for those who have suffered a broken neck, I found Sarah's book to be helpful for a back pain sufferer.

—Jennifer Fiebig

Snapped

A Helpful Guide for Broken Neck Recovery

Sarah Stockett

Printed in the United States of America

ISBN: 978-1-7336023-0-3

Library of Congress Control Number: 2019932519

23 22 21 20 19   5 4 3 2 1

Cover Design & Interior Book Design: FuzionPrint

Published by FuzionPress

1250 E 115th Street, Burnsville, MN

Table of Contents

Foreword 7

A Little Backstory 9

1. Sliding into Home 11

2. Everything You Need to Know About Your Cervical Spine.................... 21

3. The First Week After the Accident 27

4. Surviving Week 2 47

5. Summertime Blues 57

6. Offering My Hard-Earned Advice 61

7. Taking Care of Your Personal Hygiene.. 71

8. Parents and Helpful Friends... 75

9. Tips for a Good Night's Sleep with a Broken Neck........................... 79

10. 20 Reasons Why I Love My Neck Brace 83

11. Out and About... 87

12. A Month After the Accident and My St. Louis Vacation.................... 91

13. The Sex Talk... 101

14. An Unpleasant Surprise... 105

15. Dealing with Stress... 109

16. The Food Funnel... 113

17. Facing the Consequences of Bad Decisions................................... 115

18. The Beginning of Kindergarten and Changes for All of Us............... 119

19. Big News from Preschool and the Hardest Test I've Ever Taken.......... 129

20. Embrace Healing... 135

21. The Mice 137

22. Two Months Since My Fall... 139

23. The Decision to Go Sugar-Free.. 143

24. Living with a Cold and a Neck Brace 147

25. The Surprise 40th Birthday Party 151

26. My Pre- and Post-Walk Stretching Routine.................................... 157

27. Life Without My Neck Brace 171

28. What I Missed Most About Yoga Will Surprise You.......................... 175

29. My Self-Rehabilitation Process 179

30. Alternative Healing Therapies... 183

31. Physical Therapy.. 199

32. It's Been a Year Since I Broke My Neck.. 223

33. Questions & Answers from Sarah... 229

Acknowledgments 233

About the Author 235

Foreword

Neck pain, as with other forms of pain, can be debilitating. As I can attest to both personally and professionally (as a board certified pain specialist), at times pain can upend your life.

The book you are about to read is one person's perspective on the pain experience. Pain is a universal component of the human condition, yet it is uniquely and subjectively felt by each individual. It has emotional, physical, and spiritual components which can cause significant dysfunction especially if it becomes chronic.

We all know what pain is, but sometimes have a hard time describing it. Sarah, however, spells out her passage through injury and eventual recovery with vivid insights into what it feels like to experience neck pain on a very personal level. In the warp and woof of daily existence, we see how she copes with her acute traumatic injury and its aftermath.

I have known Sarah for many years now in her role as a Pilates instructor. She truly knows her stuff and is uniquely qualified to discuss her journey through adversity. She is a STOTT PILATES® Certified Instructor in Matwork, Reformer, Cadillac, Chair, and Barrels since 2007. She is also a certified yoga instructor (RYT-200), as well as a former certified personal trainer.

She gives advice that is both accurate and sensible for a (mostly) compliant patient with a stable neck injury. Her special perspective gives her a distinctive voice in telling a personal story that hopefully can help others. By reading this book, I hope you find inspiration and hope that self-motivation, choosing action, and moving forward with your life (despite what it throws at you) is a vital component to healing and recovery.

Alejandro Blachar, MD
Pain Management Physician
Mosaic Life Care
Saint Joseph, MO

A Little Backstory

When I broke my neck, it felt like a very inconvenient time for an injury. Of course, as a Pilates and yoga instructor, blogger, YouTuber, and part-time stay-at-home mom of two boys, I can say that actually *no time* would have been a "good" time for me to hurt myself.

Just months before my injury, my husband accepted a new position with odd hours. My husband is a lineman. They are the folks who turn your power back on after a storm knocks it out. In April, he accepted a new position that put him on shift work. His job switched from a Monday thru Friday 8 a.m. to 4 p.m. job to Wednesday thru Saturday 11 a.m. to 9:30 p.m.

Very shortly, the whole family fell in love with the schedule change. Although these new hours might sound inconvenient for a father of two young sons, it was actually pretty ideal because he could spend his quality time with them in the morning, join us for dinner most of the time, and help tuck them in at night (because we're night owls).

After about a month of this cushy schedule, my husband decided that he wanted to go to college to get a degree, and in May 2017, he started online classes toward an undergraduate degree. I'm very thankful that the online classes he was taking offered enough flexibility that my accident didn't get in the way of completing the courses.

Thankfully, my husband's schedule allowed for him to drop off our kids in the morning. When I broke my neck, our five-year-old went to afternoon preschool two days a week. Up until my break, the two-year-old and I would drop off his older brother and go home for a nap. Then, after a couple of hours, we would wake up and get the five-year-old from preschool. It was a polished process that didn't easily allow for the driving hiatus that happened when I broke my neck.

For the other three days of my work week, the boys went to a sitter. On these work days, I would meet one-on-one with clients in the morning and then research and write for my website in the afternoon. Sometimes, I even filmed Pilates and yoga videos for my YouTube channel.

Part of what drew me to Pilates and yoga was my passion for understanding the body and how muscles work. When I decided to get certified to teach Pilates, I picked a program that emphasized the understanding of muscles and how Pilates exercises can impact them, creating a physical therapy-type experience. I looked for a comparable program when I decided to get certified in yoga.

Although I have a great interest in anatomy and physical therapy-type exercises, I want to make it very clear that I am not a medical professional. This book is a diary-style collection of my experiences, research, and information from my own doctors or therapists.

Sliding into Home

1

S ummer is my favorite time of year. With the warm weather, increased sunlight, and my boys' sudden interest in baseball, I was prepared to maximize my outdoor time. However, one bad decision after dinner on Friday June 30, 2017 put a temporary end to my outdoor dreams.

June 30, 2017

It took forever for my older son to have *any* interest in sports. Truthfully, it wasn't until his younger brother started wanting to play baseball that he became interested. In the same week, my five-year-old and two-year-old learned to throw a ball overhand. With both of them enthusiastic about learning about and playing baseball, we took to our yard every night after dinner to play ball.

After some practice batting and throwing, I was ready to teach the basics of base running. Today, I decided to teach them how to field the ball and tag out a runner. Unfortunately, I made a huge mistake when I set up the bases.

Our house is on a hill, with no flat area where we could play. I set up the bases the best I could with second base at the top of the hill, first and third at a mid-point on the hill, and home plate downhill on the patio in front of our back door.

When I was up to bat, the boys were ready in the field. I tossed the ball up and whacked it with everything I could. I was determined to show these kids that Mom is a force to be reckoned with.

It sailed into our "outfield," and the kids scrambled to get it. I headed toward third and noticed that my older son was coming toward me, so I stopped there.

"You're out," he said tapping me with the ball.

"No, it doesn't work like that. I'm on base. You can't tag me and tell me I'm out when I'm on base."

"Well, when can I tag you?"

"Whenever I'm not on base like when I run for home."

He looked me square in the eyes. "Well, you better run, then."

It wasn't a threat as much as a challenge, and I accepted. With a glint in my eye, I took off at a dead sprint down a very steep hill.

About a third of the way down the hill, I felt like I was doing the same run that Scooby Doo does when he's not moving forward and is staying in the same place while his legs work frantically. I call it the "Scooby shuffle." Although I'm sure I wasn't there long, it felt like someone had pressed pause on my life. Time stood still long enough for me to think, "Well, *this* was a bad idea."

Then, like someone pressed play, I flailed down the hill, launched myself like a lawn dart, slid across the concrete, and head-butted my aluminum doorframe. *Don't move*, I told myself.

I hadn't passed out, and I hadn't heard a snap or crack. Those had to be good signs, right? Even when the first crimson drop splattered on the concrete in front of me, I was still optimistic. Then, I noticed that I couldn't talk. For a moment, my tongue felt like it swelled to fill my mouth. I started to moan. What came out instead was an odd, horrifying noise.

Right after my mom had her stroke, she would moan this guttural, disturbing groan when she was in pain. The noise was unlike any I'd ever heard a human make. When she would groan, it sent a pain through to my bones and scared me like no noise has ever done before.

When I heard that groan come out of my mouth, my top priority was to shut up. I didn't want my kids hearing that noise and getting scared. If I could keep it together and do all the right things, we'd make it out of this situation without a monthly therapy bill for the kids.

I closed my mouth and swallowed. I was relieved to discover that my tongue wasn't actually swollen. I took a deep breath and swallowed again. There wasn't the metallic taste of blood, which was comforting, too. Still, I knew we would be going to the hospital.

My forehead itched, and I watched another drop of blood hit the concrete beneath me. Then came another. *Stay still. Don't move.*

I heard my kids asking me if I was okay. I had to say something because they were getting worried. When I went to say, "No," it came out of my mouth like the guttural moan. I would have to do better next time if the kids were going to stay calm.

The Call

I swallowed, took a deep breath, and in an impressively calm voice, asked my five-year-old to get my phone. It was a tough decision—911 or husband? I tried to think through everything as best as I could and figured that my working husband should be the first call. When my son came out, I dialed my husband. "Tell your dad to come home."

My older son walked off with the phone while he talked to his dad. Before long, he came back and said that Dad was on his way.

Next, I sent him inside to get a paper towel. I wanted to figure out how badly my head was hurt without moving. While he was gone, I used my fingers to gently feel around to different parts of my head. Luckily, it seemed like most of my head was fine. There was a very obvious, drippy gash above my right eye, and a little bit of ooze coming down from the top of my head about where I wear the part in my hair.

By the time he came back with the paper towel, I felt confident that we wouldn't need an ambulance. I looked at my hands. My nails were broken, ripped, and jagged from my trip across about five feet of concrete as I fell.

Then, for some nonsensical reason, my fingernails became my top priority. Maybe it was because it was something I could control or maybe it's because I was trying to distract myself so I wouldn't lose my cool. I sent my two-year-old inside to get the nail trimmers, and I carefully took a seat on the back step. As I trimmed my nails, the thought hit me that it might take my husband a while to get home. I wasn't sure exactly how long I should sit on our slab. How bad was I?

I started calling people who live near me. No one answered. Friday nights in the summer everyone has plans.

Carefully, I stood up, which went well, so I stepped into the house to look at myself in the bathroom mirror. I was trying to determine whether I really should call an ambulance when I heard my husband's truck pull up. We loaded up, and all four of us went to the hospital.

The whole ride to the hospital, I held my neck, rubbing it and creating a splint of sorts with my thumbs. Nothing felt especially wrong, but I had discomfort at the base of my skull, which seemed pretty normal since I had head-butted my house.

The ER

We were very lucky. Right away, I was admitted and taken to a room. Truthfully, if our ER would have been busy that night, I might have waited for hours in the waiting room before getting treatment because I only looked banged up. I had sensation and strength in my hands and feet, I hadn't lost consciousness, and I could easily turn my head to talk to people when they spoke to me. I'm so thankful I was able to be seen immediately.

To assess my damage, the nurse asked me questions like my name and the date. She asked me what had happened. Then, she asked who the President was, and I laughed. Apparently, that was the right answer because she moved on to her final question. "Well, I have to know. Did he tag you out?"

"No, I was safe at home. Or, rather, he didn't tag me out," I answered. The last part was more correct. Given the extent of my injuries and the fact that they happened on the threshold of my home, I couldn't really say that I was *safe at home*.

In our room in the ER, the TV was on my right. I easily turned my head and my oldest snuggled up next to me while we watched one of the Shrek movies on TV.

Before too long, they sent the widest wheelchair I've ever seen to take me to my CT-scan. Once in the imaging room, I easily got up onto the table. I adjusted myself to get comfortable and didn't notice anything alarming. Truthfully, I was only concerned about swelling or bleeding in my brain.

I was afraid that I might have sustained some sort of brain injury or caused some bleeding. I didn't want to stay home from the hospital and run the risk that I might die in my sleep. After I hit my head, I knew right away that I wanted to go to the hospital and have a CT-scan done to verify that I didn't have any brain trauma.

After the test, they took me back to my room, and the technicians showed up to X-ray my knee. My knee was badly scraped from my glide across the concrete, and the doctor wanted to make sure my patellar tendon was still attached. Easily, I bent my knee and moved my leg into position. I figured all we had to do was wait for an "all clear" on the CT-scan, and we'd get to go home.

That's what my doctor thought, too. He had already talked to me about how the bumps and bruises would come out of the woodwork over the next couple of days. He even guessed that I'd need to go to the chiropractor.

"Before I go," he said, "I just have to ask—Did he tag you out?"

"No, I was safe—relatively speaking," I answered.

"Well, thank goodness for that. How terrible would it be if you fell like this *and* you got tagged out?"

"Yeah, it would have been *so* embarrassing if he tagged me out," I answered only somewhat sarcastically. In truth, beating my long-legged son in a foot race was the only silver lining I could find to my fall right now, so I proudly clung to my win.

The doctor got a good chuckle and left the room to wait for my results. At one point, the oldest child and I decided we needed to go to the bathroom. I asked the nurse if we could go, and she gave me directions. When we came back, the doctor and nurse both rushed into the room.

The Diagnosis

Apparently, while my son and I were in the bathroom, the CT-scan results came back. They showed that I had a fracture at the facet joint of my C6 up to my C5. (When you feel the back of your neck with your hand, the bony parts that you feel are the facet joints.) Fortunately, the fracture stayed perfectly aligned, and the doctor believed that I wouldn't require surgery.

"A fracture? Is that like a crack?" I asked.

"Well, it's sort of like that. You're going to need to wear this neck brace to help keep everything aligned. You'll stay overnight, and we'll have the on-call neurosurgeon see you in the morning."

He wouldn't come right out and say it. I think he knew the words would be too much of a shock.

Broken? I broke my neck? I couldn't believe it. That couldn't be right. Broken necks kill people. Or, you could go the Christopher Reeve route of being paralyzed.

When I was a kid, Superman was my favorite. I watched every Superman movie and knew who Christopher Reeve was by name—Superman. Then, he was in a horseback riding accident, broke his neck, and was paralyzed from the neck down, changing his life forever. That was it—the end of Superman.

But surely I didn't have a broken neck. The doctor must somehow be wrong.

All of a sudden, I was the center of a flurry of activity. People all around me were working quickly to get the collar on, clean my cuts, and fix my eyebrow. I thought, *This must be what Miss America feels like.*

"Do you want glue or stitches, Sarah?"

It seemed a ridiculous question. My brain screamed: *I want to go home! I don't want to have a broken neck! And you're asking whether I prefer glue or stitches?*

"Uh. Glue," I answered. The doctor and nurse trimmed my eyebrows, cleaned my wound, and glued my gash shut.

I needed to stay the night for observation. Honestly, I didn't mind. After learning that my neck was broken, I wasn't sure what kind of pain to expect. Up to that point, my pain was very quickly and easily controlled with acetaminophen. Yep, a regular dose of over-the-counter acetaminophen. It took my level-5 pain rank down to a level 1 in about 15 minutes.

Still, I worried my pain would increase through the night. Maybe the adrenaline of the accident was still pumping through me, preventing me from feeling the extent of the damage that had been done. I didn't know, and I did not want to find out.

My Room

The ER nurse, my husband, and the kids transferred me to my hospital room for the night. It was 12:30 a.m., and my kids were hanging in there. What troopers!

After I was settled in, and as soon as my family was out the door, I was flooded with a wave of emotions. Finally, the floodgates opened, and I started sobbing. The shift nurse then came in to ask more questions.

That poor nurse...I have no idea what she said. All I remember is that I couldn't stop thinking about what might have happened. What if I would have died right there in front of my children? What if I would have passed out? They would have been traumatized for forever.

Or, what if I would have been paralyzed? Our lives would have been completely changed. I think of all the what ifs, including what if I would have hit my eye (and not my eyebrow) on the piece of metal trim at the threshold to our house?

Thinking of all the other worse-yet-possible outcomes from my fall leaves my head spinning. I'm overwhelmed with horrible visions of what could have been.

Then, there is the nurse. She's asking me questions, and I suppose I'm answering them. All I remember is crying through those crappy one-ply hospital tissues as fast as she could pass them to me. For 20 minutes, she asked me questions and passed me tissues. When we finished, I was exhausted.

She adjusted me in bed, and we decided that she would come back at 1:45 a.m. to give me my next dose of acetaminophen. I was very concerned that my pain would increase, thinking: *Better to stay in front of the pain than get behind it.*

For a moment, I was fine. At least, I thought I was fine. I felt okay, took a deep breath, and completely fell apart. Panic, anger, and self-pity coursed through my veins, and I started bawling.

There's nothing I hate more than having someone mess with my plans, and the Universe was messing with my plans in a big, bad way. My whole work schedule was screwed. As a new yoga and Pilates blogger with a goal of posting once a day for a year, I saw my production schedule going up in flames. I couldn't film the videos that I relied on for three posts a week, and I couldn't teach classes.

Then, I shifted to anger. People sometimes don't give anger the credit that it deserves, but anger can be a real motivator. Anger can be the kick in the pants that you need to persevere. That's what it was for me.

I was angry that I had been foolish and let myself get hurt. I was angry that my whole summer was going to be ruined by this neck brace. I was also extremely angry that some unseen force was messing with my work schedule. Nothing was going to get in the way of my publishing schedule. I vowed that I would look over what needed to be done and make changes. The largest change would be my posts on Saturdays, the Weekend Workout. Those posts were 20–30 minute workout videos. Obviously, I wasn't going to be doing that for a while with my broken neck.

I had an idea. I decided to write about my broken-neck experience and share any thoughts or tips I discovered along the way. Resolved and content, I dozed off.

Day Shift

Through the night, I slept in short stretches. Periodically, nurses would pop in to check on me. It was always very comforting to me that: 1) I woke up each time they came in, 2) I still knew my name and birthday, and 3) My pain level was very tolerable.

Luckily for me, the doctor and neurosurgeon liked to make their rounds early, and I might be one of the first visits they made. My neurosurgeon was the first one to visit. He checked my strength and the sensations in my hands and feet, and he concluded that I needed to wear my neck brace at all times, except when in the shower. I couldn't believe that I would potentially have a brief respite from wearing the neck brace while in the shower. However, isn't the shower one of the most common places where people slip, fall, and break their neck? Couldn't a new fall without my neck brace mean death or paralysis?

The idea of being brace-free simultaneously excited and frightened me. The on-call doctor came through, and I kid you not, by 10:30 a.m., I was ready to go home.

My husband and kids, however, were still working on eating breakfast and getting dressed. I ordered my breakfast and started watching some TV. I was restless and ready to leave. I couldn't find anything on TV to keep my attention, so I turned it off and rested.

By the time we left, I was exhausted. My family took me home. I notified family and friends of my accident, crawled into bed, and slept. I did not even wake myself up to take more acetaminophen.

Everything You Need to Know About Your Cervical Spine

2

It's possible you don't know much about the structure of your neck, which is also known as the cervical spine. Even as a Pilates and yoga instructor who has studied anatomy for years, my knowledge was very limited. Because clients had neck problems, I had learned a little bit about what might be impacting them. However, it wasn't until I broke my neck that I became extremely interested in the cervical spine.

Your Cervical Vertebrae

You have 7 cervical vertebrae. Your very first vertebra is known as C1, and it's also called the *atlas*. According to Wikipedia ([https://en.wikipedia.org/wiki/Atlas_(anatomy)], it is so named because, like the mythological legend Atlas, it is carrying a great weight. Unlike the legend, your atlas is carrying the weight of your skull and not the Earth.

This is an image of my atlas.

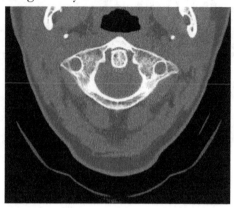

Just below your atlas is your second vertebra (C2), which is called the *axis*." This is because the axis is the pivot point that helps the skull and atlas turn when you look from side to side. These top two cervical vertebrae are shaped slightly differently from each other and from the lower cervical vertebrae because their functions differ.

None of the other vertebrae have fun names, but that doesn't mean they're not important. These lower cervical vertebrae are responsible for supporting the head and neck, protecting the spinal cord, and creating space and structure for nerves and blood vessels.

This is an image of my C4.

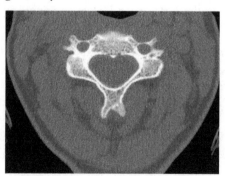

In the middle of each vertebrae is a rather large space for the spinal cord to pass through. To the left and right sides, there are little grooves and holes in the bone to allow for nerves and blood vessels. The nerves come off the spinal cord and serve as a network for communication with the upper body.

Nerves From the Cervical Spine

The nerves that come directly off the spinal cord are named in conjunction with the vertebra beneath them. For example, the C7 nerve comes off the spinal cord above the C7 vertebra and passes through the C6-C7 neural foramen. (The foramen is the opening between vertebrae through which nerves pass.)

Since there are only 7 cervical vertebrae, it might seem odd to see a C8 nerve listed. The C8 nerve exits between C7 and T1. It still works with the other cervical spine nerves, which is why it's listed as C8 and not T1.

Cervical Nerves

According to an article used with permission, written by Paul J. Slosar, MD and published by Veritas Health at Spine-Health.com (https://www.spine-health.com/conditions/spine-anatomy/cervical-nerves), here are the duties of the nerves at each vertebra:

- C1 (Atlas) controls movements of the head and neck, including forward, backward, and sideways movements.
- C2 (Axis) controls movements of the head and neck, including forward, backward, and sideways movements. It is also responsible for sensation on the top of the head.

- C3 controls movements of the head and neck, including forward, backward, and sideways movements. It is also responsible for sensation on the side of the face and on the back of the head.
- C4 "helps control the shoulders as well as the diaphragm." This nerve greatly impacts breathing.
- C5 controls the muscles in your shoulders, upper arm, and possibly forearm. This includes the deltoids and biceps.
- C6 controls the wrist extensors and also can feed into the biceps. The area covered starts at "the top of the shoulders and runs down the side of the arm and into the thumb side of the hand."
- C7 controls the triceps and runs from "the shoulder down the back of the arm and into the middle finger."
- C8 controls the hands and "covers the lower part of the shoulder and goes down the arm into the pinky side of the hand."

As you can see, the nerves that come from the cervical spine impact your sensation in your head, neck, diaphragm, shoulders, arms, and hands. The nerves send messages to the muscles in these parts of your body. Unfortunately, sometimes tight muscles connected to the spine can impact the quality or the content of the messages being sent.

Muscles That Impact the Cervical Spine

Your brain has something it wants your left hand to do. It sends a message down, through the spinal cord, out through the appropriate nerve root, and the message goes to the left hand.

What if you have a vertebra out of place, slightly compressing the nerve root?

Unfortunately, the message gets relayed more like a game of telephone. Sure, the message might come out as intended. However, it may become garbled along the way.

Muscles That Impact the Neck

Because of this, it's important to know which muscles connect to the cervical spine. This is a list of all the muscles that connect to any portion of the cervical vertebrae. I learned all of the following information when I was studying to become a certified Pilates instructor.

- **Levator Scapulae:** Levator scapulae originates on C1–C4. It helps lift your scapula (shoulder blade) and, by working the opposite way, helps lower your ear toward your shoulder.
- **Rhomboid Minor:** Rhomboid minor originates on C7 and T1. Its primary job is to retract and elevate the scapula.
- **Scalenes**: The anterior scalenes originate on C3-C6, the medial scalenes originate on C2–C7, and the posterior scalenes originate on C4-C6. Scalenes help you bring your ear toward the shoulder of the working muscle and turn your head away from the working muscle.
- **Spinal Muscles:** Spinal muscles run all up and down your spine. It's safe to say that each cervical vertebra has several spinal muscles connected to it. These spinal muscles help you keep a neutral spine, extend it, rotate it, and flex it to the side.
- **Sternocleidomastoid:** This muscle inserts on the base of your skull. Sternocleidomastoid helps you bring your ear

toward the shoulder of the working muscle and turns your head away from the working muscle.

- **Upper Trapezius:** The upper trapezius originates at the base of the skull and on C7. Primarily, the upper trapezius elevates the scapula like when you're shrugging your shoulder.

What Do I Do With This Information?

Now you know approximately which nerves from your cervical spine are responsible for which muscles or areas of your upper body. Whether you have a broken neck or not, this information is valuable because it can help you know what to do if you have pain or an odd sensation.

For those with a broken neck, this information can work like a trip to the fortuneteller. Check out the lists to see what muscles and nerves are on or near your broken vertebra. It's a safe bet that you will have issues with these muscles and nerves when you're finally healed and ready to resume normal activity.

The First Week
After the Accident

3

After I was released from the hospital in the morning, I began the dreaded task—notification of family and friends. In particular, I did not want to tell my parents. I was certain Mom would get upset when she learned of my broken neck.

This is probably because I was still internally freaking out about it. For many people, a broken neck means instant death. For others, it means a lifetime of disability. But for me, it only meant a neck brace.

The relative lack of damage, the

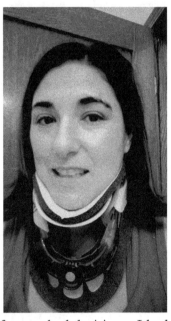

escape of a lifetime of consequences for one bad decision—I had no idea why I was this lucky when many others were not. I was most grateful that I had limited damage from my fall.

I made my way upstairs to my bed, propped myself up, and grabbed my phone. I looked at it. A black screen reflected back to me some banged-up woman with a neck brace. I took a deep breath and dialed my mom's cell phone.

When Dad answered, I was relieved. "Hey, Dad. Is Mom there?"

"Well, yes, but she's getting her haircut."

"Oh good!" I could pass off the role of bad news messenger to my dad. "Hey, I need to tell you something, and I need you to stay calm. Don't freak out or anything, and don't say anything that would make Mom think that there's a problem, okay?"

"Okay, Sarah…"

"I fell last night and fractured my neck, but I'm alright. I'm at home, and I have to wear a neck brace for eight weeks to three months. I'm worried Mom will get upset. Will you tell her when you guys are in the car?"

"Sure. What were you doing?" I told him the story and, when I got to the end, he asked, "Well, did he tag you out?"

"No, thank you, I can out-run a five-year-old, Dad."

"Well, thank goodness for that. Otherwise, this would have been really embarrassing."

"Thanks, Dad."

"I love you, Sarah. I'm glad you're okay. I'll let your mom know."

I ate some lunch and about the time I finished, Mom and Dad called. Mom handled the news amazingly well and wasn't upset at all. She suggested that she and Dad come to help with the boys.

I was quite relieved. I absolutely wanted their help, plus I wanted to see them. We had planned a family trip to go to St. Louis to celebrate the Fourth of July. Sunday morning, once my husband was off work, we were supposed to head out. I wanted to watch glorious fireworks displays with them and hopefully give my boys some of the memories that I had as a kid watching large, county fireworks displays. Instead, we would celebrate at home where I broke my neck a handful of days ago, watching fireworks from my driveway—the scene of the crime.

My trip wasn't the only Fourth of July festivity I had to cancel. It was time for my second-most unhappy notification of the day— I let my friends know why the boys and I wouldn't be making it out to their Fourth of July party today.

Since it's a Saturday, my husband would have been working, but the boys and I planned to go to the party. We love parties. Plus, my friend tends to go all-out for this celebration. She hires a band and has carnival rides and ponies. This celebration is a big one for her, and I couldn't wait to be part of the fun with the boys.

I really hated to miss out. I hate having to cancel any commitments I make, I hate not getting to see my friends, and I hate not getting to see my boys have fun. It drives me nuts to think of other people laughing and doing fun things while I do…whatever. Missing out makes me grumpy.

Then, come the flood of "Oh my gosh! Let me know if you need anything!" texts. I know these women friends mean it, and it makes me feel like George Bailey in *It's a Wonderful Life* when all his friends show up to help him at the end of the movie. I'm touched and appreciative of their generous, kind offers and genuine concern. I start to cry happy tears, knowing that I'm so loved. Finally, I decide to make my injury Facebook-official and then take a nap.

I slept four hours. The nap felt amazing. My bed was much more comfortable than the hospital bed and, as the daylight filled my room, I felt warm and optimistic. I do love napping when it's light outside.

When I woke up, I gathered all the courage I could muster and decided to try taking a bath. I was petrified. First, I would have to figure out how to get my tank top off while wearing a neck brace. Then, I would have to remove my sports bra. My first thought was scissors, but I ended up using my patience. Scissors were a viable second option, though.

On top of all of that, I would have to remove the bandages covering my right knee and left foot and clean whatever carnage was beneath them. Then, there would be the whole rebandaging process. Thankfully, my husband went to the store and bought giant bandages, antiseptic, and antibiotic cream. I was not excited to discover how my completely ripped-open knee and scraped foot would feel when hot water and soap hit them.

Once I was ready to get in the tub, I was extremely conflicted. On one hand, the doctor told me that I could take the neck brace off for bathing. On the other hand, this thing was keeping a part of my spine in place—something that meant that I wouldn't have to live with a lifetime of paralysis or (worse yet) death.

I tried to talk myself into removing the neck brace, but I simply couldn't. I was too afraid. Instead, I sat upright in the tub and used a washcloth to clean myself.

It was actually comforting to sit in the warm water, and my wounds didn't sting at all. I took a deep breath. Each time I do something scary and new, I will remind myself that this is one of the many steps to a full recovery. *I can do this.*

With a clean body and the confidence that comes with completing a dreaded task, I decided to write. If my writing schedule was going to be derailed by this accident, I was going to take full advantage of it. I decided to do my best to write about my experiences with the hope that I would be able to help someone else in a similar situation. Maybe, at the end of all of this, I might even have enough for a whole book.

My fingers were twitching with excitement, and my body was filled with acetaminophen. I started writing. When you're beginning a long journey, what better way to start than with some goals.

Goals for a Complete Recovery

1. Don't move your head.
2. Keep your body strong so you don't mess up the rest of your spine.
3. Sleep/rest a lot.
4. Figure out how to keep your life kind of status quo.
5. Remember—always move with intention. Engage your abdominal muscles (abs) before you do *anything*. In the case of any spinal injury, it is always a possibility that your present injury can lead to an additional injury in another part of the spine.
6. After spending 15 years in fitness, I was more than aware how one injury could lead to another, sometimes larger, injury. My neck injury is sufficient, and my plan is to be as smart and mindful as I can be when I move so that I don't end up accidentally giving myself a greater injury. Although I can't actually do anything to speed up my recovery, I can do my best to not injure myself further.

Random Thoughts for the Day

1. Wear the cervical collar and drink lots of milk and water. The faster I can get this fracture to heal, the faster I can be out of this collar. If I do what I'm supposed to, maybe I can be out of this thing at my eight-week checkup.
2. The road rash on my scalp and knee are the most uncomfortable part of this whole situation, but they should heal in maybe a week.
3. I have a real goose egg where they had to glue my face shut, which is also very uncomfortable.

4. Maybe I'll take this week off work. It seems deserved. Plus, I've already scheduled my posts for the next month. One week off won't put me too far behind.

5. Hey, this cervical collar will give me the neutral cervical spine that I've been trying to achieve for years. Pre-accident, I was at the chiropractor's office about every week because some of my neck muscles (particularly the scalenes, sternocleidomastoid, and upper trapezius) were tight and would tense, pulling my neck out of place. No matter what I tried, they seemed to always defeat me and pull the vertebrae in my neck askew. With this brace, I have the upper hand, and I might actually win this battle.

   In the meantime, my upper back hates me right now for the postural changes that we're making. It hates the new constantly-neutral position of my head and neck, and it longs for the good old days with my poor posture. That's not going to happen. My upper back hurts, and I'm in pain. Take deep breaths. It's all part of the process.

6. Use as many other body parts to help you as you can. In particular, use your forearms and hands to help you get settled in bed. Look for other ways to use your hands, arms, legs, and feet to help adjust and get comfortable.

7. Take each day as it comes. This is all a process. Remember, this too shall pass.

July 2, 2017

I've never been hit by a bus, but I imagine this might be what it feels like. My head hurts all over, the collar seems to be digging into my skull, and sitting upright is exhausting. Overall, I'll probably spend more time horizontal than upright.

I'm most thankful that it's Sunday and my husband is at home. He took off work yesterday to take care of the boys, and he's taking care of them now while I rest. They're all doing a good job of balancing letting me rest and involving me in their day. That can't be easy.

I found a new way to bandage my knee, and now it hurts less when I bend it. Truthfully, I was lucky because part of my knee was healing already. A small part about a quarter of an inch from the top of the wound closed. It was the oddest thing to have a narrow strip healing, separating the wound into two distinct sections. This provided an opportunity for some creative bandaging. I could use a small strip over the top wound and then a medium-sized bandage over the larger portion of my knee. It worked, and I was finally able to bend it better.

Also, I think that my knee is getting its range of motion back. Happily, I no longer have to hike my right hip up to my ribs in order to take a step on the stairs.

Aside from these gains, my pain today is much worse. The whole time I was awake, I took acetaminophen every four hours. The end result was that my head hurt less, but my stomach was a mess. Tomorrow, I will try to take less acetaminophen. Hopefully, a good night's sleep will bring a better tomorrow.

July 3, 2017

Okay. Today's the day. I have to shower. My hair is very gross, and I became a little sweaty yesterday, so...yeah. It's time to shower.

I'm stalling. Right now, I'm supposed to be showering, but instead, I'm discovering other things that are imperative to complete before tackling the task at hand. I've closed out the month of June for my business, written my journal entries for July

1 and 2, and started on July 3—all because I don't want to stand in the shower without a neck brace.

I'm terrified. This thing, this neck brace, is what separates me from all the people who have died from a broken neck. This brace is the one difference that we have to our stories. Yet, one slip in the shower, one wrong movement, and I could join them for forever. People slip and break their necks in a shower, and I should not be doing this. I should not shower without the brace.

The doctor is the trusted medical professional, and he said I should shower without it. Ugh! I know I have to do this. I have to shower. I'm going to shower. God help me.

I did it! And, like many things in life, it was not near as difficult as I thought it would be. It didn't hurt at all when I washed the road rash on my scalp. My face, however, was quite the opposite.

The pressure from the showerhead was enough to set the right side of my face prickling with pain. Then, when I gently washed my face, it burned, alerting me that my face is a work in progress.

On the other hand, every day my foot and knee ooze out less goo. I haven't had to take as much acetaminophen. Plus, my right knee is bending better, making it easier to get up and down the stairs. All of these are pretty significant wins.

I haven't mentioned this, but I think I jammed my three center fingers on my left hand. They have been sore at the top joints since the day after my fall. Honestly, at first, I thought I was imagining the discomfort. Then, I remembered that I had completely broken the nails on those three fingers in the fall.

I remember sending the little one into the house to get me nail trimmers while we waited for help. Calmly, I trimmed all the nails on my left hand, and then contemplated whether I should do my right. *Who* does that?! Blood is coming out of my head, and my instinct is to trim my fingernails? That's crazy! However, I *did not* want to go to the hospital with jagged fingernails or only one trimmed hand. The only logical choice was to perform the oddest manicure I've ever had.

Mastering the Brace

Aside from the shower, my other goal for the day is to learn how to adjust my neck brace. Right now, I think it is adjusted correctly, but I want to know how to adjust it so that I can take my care into my own hands.

The brace is pretty cool; it's an Aspen Vista. It's two pieces with Velcro straps and a circle knob on the front. If I pull the knob out and rotate, it will make the chin support raise or lower. My chin support was set by the doctor, so I think it's where I want it to be.

Here's how I put on my neck brace:

1. Get the front part of my collar placed correctly under my chin.
2. Place a very slight amount of pressure on the chin rest to help hold it in place.
3. Lift my hair off the back of my neck. I use a hair clip or pony tail holder to help.
4. Place the back part of the brace in the correct spot behind my neck.
5. Gently tuck the front edges of the front piece into the back piece to ensure the brace is not too loose on my neck.
6. Fasten the Velcro straps.

*****

I'll get lots of practice taking off and putting on the brace. Unfortunately, I discovered that my excellent shampoo job did not wash all of the antibiotic cream from the hospital off my scalp. This means I still have an oil slick in the middle of my head. I see another shower in my near future.

The Update: Four Days After My Fall

- **Head**: On the upside, the swelling is going down in the knot on my head. Unfortunately, this makes that spot hurt quite a bit. I can see a yellow-green line appear under my right eye—the first signs of a black eye that's already healing. The road rash on my scalp is doing well and has started scabbing and rubbing off. My scalp is very greasy where they used the antibiotic cream. I think that this is helpful to the scab there.
- **Neck**: Yup, still broken. Still uncomfortable.
- **Shoulders**: Happily, the tetanus shot has been absorbed into my system, and I can raise my right arm easily now. However, I'm still having some pain on the back of my right shoulder. No bruising, but it's still sensitive to the touch on the farthest point of my shoulder blade. How the heck did that happen?
- **Elbows**: The pain in my elbow crease continues, marking where the IV port was. I'm no stranger to IVs, but I've never had pain like this for days after the removal.
- **Fingers**: My pointer finger is quite a bit better, but I still feel like my middle and ring fingers are jammed at the farthest joint.

- **Thighs**: The bruise on my left thigh is now bigger than the palm of my hand. It's yellow, purple, blue, and green. Honestly, I think it will be gone in a couple of days.
- **Knees**: The right knee is still gooey, but it's definitely less than yesterday.
- **Feet**: The top of my left foot is healing well. I spent a good amount of time today with the bandage off, hoping that the air will help it scab up.

July 4, 2017

Last night, I slept very poorly. I'm not sure if it was because of how I was positioned in bed or maybe how I put the neck brace on after my shower, but I felt the plastic frame of the brace pressing into the back of my skull. This made me worry that maybe I would have to sleep this way for the next few weeks.

There seem to be two settings to this neck brace. I can have the plastic smash into the back of my skull or I can shift the brace and have it apply pressure to the bottom of my ears, similar to having something try to slide my ears up my head. Either way, I don't like those choices.

Our holiday together was a lot less eventful than usual, but it was enjoyable nonetheless. Then, our neighbors started shooting off fireworks. We grabbed lawn chairs and sat in the driveway, watching our neighborhood display. My younger son was very excited that he could sit outside in his pajamas and watch the night sky light up.

Celebrating with the family was the pick-me-up that I needed. When you see the world through a child's eyes, it's a lot easier to forget about your pain and feel thankful for how blessed you've been.

Then, I went to bed, took some acetaminophen, positioned myself, and for the first time all night, I was comfortable. Mind you, it wasn't simply that I wasn't uncomfortable; *I was comfortable.* Thankfully, I slept for several hours before the sun and my kids woke me up.

Meditation for Pain Management

I'm not one to sit around and take acetaminophen for my pain. On my website, I'm used to giving people advice on Pilates exercises and yoga poses they can do to help relieve their pain. Now, I'm sitting here, totally unable to exercise, and in a world of pain.

I tried to rest. Pain. I took medicine. Pain.

My options felt very limited. Then, it hit me—meditation. Meditation is an important component of yoga, and all you have to do is rest in a comfortable position. I decided to give it my best shot to create a meditation for pain relief.

Meditation for pain management is very common. One of my friends with rheumatoid arthritis took a class at the Mayo Clinic specifically geared to relaxation as a pain-management tool. She found the information there very valuable. I wish I had her handbook, but I didn't. Here's what I created instead.

My Meditation

Some people like to be seated on the floor, but I prefer to be on my back in bed.

Close your eyes. Imagine your body is a raised garden bed. Pieces of wood outline your body and keep your greenery contained.

Imagine looking at your garden. Understand that everything within the garden correlates directly to what is within you. Study the plants and the growth. Do you see any empty spots? Do you see different plants?

Now, see yourself as a gardener approaching the garden bed.

As you meditate, the garden is your body, the gardener is your mind, and your spirit is reflected as the observer. Watch your gardener observe the garden. Notice how your gardener knows exactly where to go to root out the cause of your **pain**. As the gardener locates weeds in your garden, watch as he/she twirls the weed around his/her hand and deliberately removes the plant. Feel the relief in your body as the gardener removes a source of pain.

Notice how the garden and gardener seem to communicate with each other. See how the gardener may start to remove a weed, stop, and readjust to grasp more appropriately. When the garden and gardener communicate, they can work together to find the true source of the issue.

As the gardener works, allow yourself to relax and feel the relief of pain leaving your boday.

July 5, 2017

I haven't mentioned this before, but falling asleep is quite a challenge. First, you have to get yourself settled in a way that you're not in any serious pain. At this point in time, *discomfort is acceptable, but pain is a deal-breaker.* This step doesn't actually take as long as you may think. If you practice meditation, it can be anywhere from one to ten minutes.

Next, you start to fall asleep and, as you doze, you think that your head is moving, which makes you freak out and wake yourself up. Your eyes snap open to find that you're looking at the exact same spot on your ceiling as when you fell asleep, and you close your eyes again, reassured that your neck is stabilized, and you're safe.

Then, comes the hard part. You fall asleep. At first, your dreams are fine. Maybe some weird stuff happens, but there's nothing scary enough that would wake you up. Gradually, things shift, and before you know it, you're reliving your accident. Every bad decision, every mistake and misstep is highlighted.

You're forced to watch and relive. All the panic and dread flood over you as you watch drops of blood slowly spat on the concrete in front of you. Your boys speak to you, asking you if you're okay. You try very hard to move your thick tongue into words, but all that comes out is a guttural, animalistic groan.

The world spins. Everything vanishes, and you're in your room. For a minute, you can't tell if you've just had a nightmare, imagining every horrible detail of some fictional accident—but then you feel the security of your cervical collar and know that it's real.

*****

Today was my husband's first day back to work. His coworkers are all kind. They asked about me, and told him that if we needed anything, we should let them know. When he told me that everyone had asked about me, it made me tear up. I truly appreciate everyone's kind thoughts and words.

July 6, 2017

Last night, I slept quite well. With much apprehension, I took my second shower. It went better than my first, and I made sure to wash a little better where the road rash is on my scalp. I didn't want to have that gooey antibiotic cream smear down the middle of my scalp after my *second* shower. It was bad enough that it stayed after my first.

Then, when I went to bed, I immediately found a comfortable position. I had no pain, no bad dreams, nothing. Only comfort and sleep, and it was everything I remembered it to be.

*****

Yesterday, my parents arrived to help me out. It's always great to have my folks around. I love watching them play with the kids. However, I hate that a majority of their visits are to help me recuperate.

Last year, they were here to help out after I had my umbilical hernia repaired. Now, here they are to help out with my broken neck. They should visit more when I'm healthy—of course, I have to get back to being healthy first.

When my folks are here, my usual workday productivity on business projects decreases. Tomorrow, I will try to work on my writing before they come over. Even though they are here to help me, I still feel good enough to have the need to play hostess. This is the exact opposite of their intention, I know, but I can't override the inert feeling to get them water or snacks.

*****

Today, my next biggest fear happened: the first sneeze. Not surprisingly, like all my other fears, it was all a lot of emotion around a very minimal activity. The sneeze was so small and polite that I bet many people wouldn't even have heard it. Thankfully, it had no impact on my neck or back.

The second sneeze was a slightly different story. It had been hours after the first sneeze, and I was feeling confident. I felt the sneeze start building in my face. *We got this,* my body told my brain. Something was off, and I ended up feeling a jolt in my spine. It wasn't anything terrible, but it was enough that I wanted to take a break to rest my back.

By the time the third sneeze came around, I had no idea what to expect. Thankfully, it was similar to my initial delicate sneeze. Now might be a good time to mention that I'm allergic to cats, and we have three indoor cats. No matter the season, I tend to do a lot of sneezing.

*****

The five-year-old returned to afternoon preschool today. Suffice to say, his teachers were pretty surprised that I broke my neck over the weekend. I'm going to bet his holiday adventures were the most interesting in his class.

*****

When I look at the colorful bruise on my leg, I see the individual colors and am reminded how much I have always loved rainbows. My eyes pick and sort through the colors, finding all my favorites. The purplish blue reminds me of the night sky after a perfect sunset. Then, it hits me that I'm looking at the largest, most painful bruise that I've ever had—a bruise that reminds me of my horrible fall and broken neck. All the positive emotions from looking at this rainbow dissolve and are replaced with anger and disgust.

This healing process has been much different than any other that I've been through before. It's a little bit of a complex ride when you have done something stupid that you have to acknowledge on a day-by-day, hour-by-hour, minute-by-minute basis because almost everything you do leaves you in pain. This is nothing like recovering from a C-section or having your umbilical hernia repaired. You are in this position because of one bad decision you made.

It's not that I'm not aware of how lucky I was. I am. It's not that I'm not grateful for escaping with such relatively minimal injuries. I am. Still, it doesn't change the fact that for the first week after my fall, I was in a lot of bad pain and was able to marginally sleep for only a few hours at a time. Psychologically, that takes a tremendous toll on a person.

Plus, there's the nightmares that you have when you do fall asleep—all the what-ifs or the slo-mo replay of your fall with a step-by-step criticism of what you could have done differently. Then, you mix all of that with the fact that I'm a very social person who gets her joy by being active and being around other people— and now I'm sequestered in my own home. If I were somehow in my own personal Inferno, this would be one of my rings of hell. Mind you, it wouldn't be the worst level, but it wouldn't be the easiest level either.

July 7, 2017

Today, I'm going back to work. Thankfully, I only have two clients today. As I write this, I have already met with them, and we all lived to tell the tale.

I am probably more tired than usual, but I did have to get up early and work. Tonight, I will sleep well; and this afternoon, I will try to take a break and rest.

It's funny. At the time, I was very enthusiastic about writing a book about the accident, but now I want to nap. Nap and watch *Cheers*.

A couple of days ago, Mom and I discovered that I have digital access to some old TV shows, such as *Cheers*. If you haven't watched *Cheers* in a while and you don't have pain when you laugh, I highly recommend that you give it a try.

Also, today marks the one-week anniversary of my big crash. One week down, possibly 12 more to go. I've decided to start thinking of my relationship with the neck brace as being similar to pregnancy, which I have also endured during summertime heat, twice. Anyway, unlike pregnancy, I will feel better and better as the days go on, *and at the end of 13 mere weeks*, I'm done! The brace comes off, therapy begins, and my life can get back to normal.

Plus, and I hope I'm not jinxing myself here, but there is a possibility that the neck brace may be able to come off earlier. Maybe I am having an eight-week relationship with this thing. Who knows? That reminds me—time for milk.

*****

The itching has started. I knew that the healing process for my face and scalp would probably be the most uncomfortable part of recovery. Well, here we are. Last night, I felt my hands creep to my scalp, looking for any unnecessary scabs to flick away. My fingers kept busy.

Then, in the middle of the night, my brain sent that message. *Ooh! What's that by your eye? Scratch it!* Since I was asleep, the rest of my body complied. You know what it was? Glue. On my eyebrow. Holding my face shut. And it hurt horribly when I tried to scratch it.

This morning, I'm pretty sure the rest of my body is still angry with that part of my brain that told me to scratch. Suffice to say, there will be no scratching of the eyebrow in the near future.

Surviving Week 2

4

July 8, 2017

Every day, my parents come over to the house from their hotel to help me out. I appreciate how helpful they have been driving me around, but my favorite part about having them here is watching how much my kids love my folks. They all joke and play together, and it warms my heart to sit back and watch them interact.

Because our day was too busy, we decided to take advantage of the hotel pool at night. After dinner, we all loaded into my car because it has enough room for all of us. Dad drove us to their hotel. We went to their room, the kids changed, and then Dad realized he had left his swim trunks in his car, which was at my house.

As it was, we had only about an hour for the kids to swim, and Dad had to improvise. He found a pair of cotton shorts and prepared to brave it into the pool with two young swimmers. Thankfully, the pool was not terribly busy.

They splashed and played. The two-year-old became independent, and he kicked away from my dad. I sat in a chair on the side. My leg wounds are still too significant for swimming in a public pool.

At the end of the night, my heart felt full. It was a perfect day.

July 9, 2017

The glue in my eyebrow started peeling. Is it because some oils I used helped dissolve the glue? In any case, after using the product on my cut, the glue started to feel tacky and gummy. I rolled it between my fingers to try to free my individual eyebrow hairs. However, I still managed to accidentally remove a few small hairs each time I pulled a gob of glue from my face.

When I finished, the top part of my gash was visible. It looks like it healed up quite well. There's a dented pink line that drops down into my eyebrow. I wonder when the rest of the glue will be ready to come off?

*****

Today, my parents left to go back home, and I was sad to see them leave. On their way out of town, they dropped me off at the yoga studio where I usually taught and also took yoga classes. I sat in on a teacher training class on loops and spirals. Physically, I was uncomfortable. Emotionally, I was grumpy. It was hard to focus and absorb any quality information.

I know no one wants to make me feel self-conscious, but we started the day by talking about my broken neck. The attention makes me feel like the main attraction at a freak show. And, although I know everyone was focused on the teacher, I still felt like people were staring at me.

Sitting up against the wall, I took deep breaths. *They're not looking at you. They're not looking at you,* I told myself over and over. I would believe it some time, right?

When the class ended, one of my friends from teacher training gave me a ride home. It was very nice to be able to talk to her and find out what was going on in her life. Right now, I've had enough drama in my life that it's such a relief to hear about other peoples' lives.

July 10, 2017

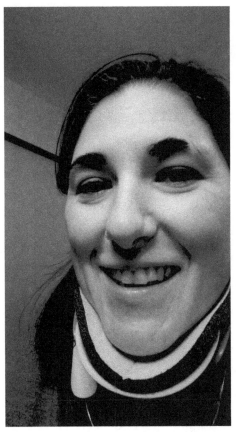

Today, I started rocking my 1990s Vanilla Ice look. With half of my right eyebrow on my face and the other half in the trashcan, I felt a little naked. Although the glue started peeling and made me think it would ball up and slide off my eyebrow, that wasn't what happened. Instead, the glue in my eyebrow was adamant about staying on each individual hair.

I tried to break it into balls and remove it bit by bit, but it would only lift a smidge away from my skin. Then, it wouldn't budge. Unfortunately, this meant that I could either pull the gobs of glue (with the eyebrows stuck to it) and essentially self-wax off half my eyebrow, or I could carefully trim it and pray that enough eyebrow hairs were left to help me look more normal.

Still, despite my best efforts, I ended up with one-and-a-half eyebrows. Honestly, no one even looks at your eyebrows when you're wearing a neck brace, but I've been doing my best to try to reduce my drastic appearance. I can only imagine the shock and *oh, that must've hurt* thoughts people have because I feel them every time I look in a mirror.

Also, today I went to my gynecologist. They were incredibly surprised not just by my appearance, but by the fact that I even showed up. I would have preferred to cancel, but gynecology appointments are scheduled about seven months out, and I didn't want to risk it and lose my sweet summertime appointment slot.

July 11, 2017

I'm not completely sure what happened. I went to bed at a pretty good time, slept until 9:30, but I'm extremely exhausted. I feel like a zombie, going through the motions without any real thought behind my actions. All day, I've been fighting fatigue, which makes me wonder—should I go to sleep or carry on this way?

Of course, staying awake is much more productive than being asleep. However, as I'm writing my entry for tonight, I can't miss noticing how *utterly exhausted* I am. Earlier this evening, I took my shower. I take my shower before the kids do now because my shower can easily take an hour from start to finish *if* I stay on task and no one bothers me.

With my shower complete, I was applying lotion and getting dressed when a thought hit me. *Here I am on day 11 and every day I take a shower and wash my hair, it feels like the most substantial thing I accomplished all day—a shower where I didn't further injure or accidentally kill myself.*

Each time I take a shower, I have that fear that I'll forget and tip my head up, or that I'll slip on something, and that will be the end of this happy healing process, and maybe even the end of me entirely.

I am petrified of this short time without my neck brace. I fully realize that I was extremely lucky with my accident. With no paralysis and no surgery to put my spine back together, I couldn't dream of asking for more than that. Still, every time I have to take my neck brace off to bathe, I ask God for just a little more. "Please, God, don't let me do something stupid and die in the shower today."

July 12, 2017

My husband dropped the boys off, which allowed me to see a client this morning. He works from 11 a.m. to 9:30 p.m. Wednesdays through Saturdays. This offers some very valuable flexibility in the morning and on Mondays and Tuesdays. In particular, I love his schedule because it allows him to drop the boys off Monday, Wednesday, and Friday mornings at daycare, take our oldest to afternoon preschool on Tuesdays, and then pick everyone up Mondays and Tuesdays. This means that I won't need to figure out a way to bum a ride from someone on these days in order to collect my children.

Then, after seeing clients and writing, I decided to take a little nap. I had a sneezing fit pre-nap today. When I say "sneezing fit," I'm not talking about two or three "ah-choos" in a row. I'm talking about six or more "ah-bwazahs"—the kind of sneezes to knock your socks off or make you wet your pants a little.

Right when I started to relax, I felt the sneezes build, and I did my best to be ready. Fortunately, I was on my back. This helped me discover: *The best way to sneeze in a neck brace is on your back.* After sneezing while sitting, standing, and bent forward; this is hands down the most comfortable way to sneeze.

When I woke up from my nap, I wrote for a little longer and got ready to pick up the boys. My friend came over to drive me to pick up the kids—my first chauffeuring experience from a friend.

I feel awkward having someone come over to my house to drive me around in my own car, but it's the best way to pick up the boys. And, with my husband at work, I don't have any other options. I'm eternally grateful for the friends and family that have already committed to interrupt their days to come over and help me make it through mine.

After picking up the boys, I wrote some more while I was making dinner. My husband was at work the whole time except for a brief window during my afternoon nap. This was my first day without my parents or my husband at home with me.

After we picked up the kids, my friend went home. Then, the kids and I enjoyed the whole evening watching TV together, playing Minecraft, then getting ready for bed. All of this happened without incident. Sometimes, I think that they especially try to do well when it's only the three of us because they feel bad for my broken neck.

That's fine. I hope they keep it up—at least until I'm cleared to live without the brace.

July 13, 2017

Holy cow! I'm not sure if I'm staying up too late at night journaling about my days or if healing truly requires quite a bit more sleep, but I woke up at 8:30 after sleeping for 9.5 hours. However, after eating breakfast, I already was spent. Seriously, I took a 30-minute siesta before my husband went to work.

This week has been a challenge because I'm sleepy and also, I'm completely relying on other people to drive me. Plus, my husband is getting ready for finals for his online college classes that he's taking. I truly miss being able to drive myself to pick up the kids or go get groceries—but I really, really miss fast food.

I love fast food, and my husband hates it. Pretty regularly, one of our dinners was pizza. Sometimes that would even fall on the day when the boys and I would hit a drive-thru for lunch.

Right now, I want ice cream in the worst way. My favorite ice cream shop is only a couple blocks from our house. It seems particularly cruel that it's close but still too far to walk. Even if the kids were bigger, it would be too far to walk there, especially in the middle of summer. I try not to obsess about it, but I admit that I'm already trying to find ways or reasons for my friends to drive me there next week when we're running errands.

Today, I have a play date with one of my very favorite friends, and she has a two-month-old. We met when our oldest kids were in music class together. They are still good friends, and I find our play dates invaluable in terms of restoring my cool and boosting my spirits. Even if I didn't feel bummed out, spending time with this friend always lifts me up.

As expected, we have a wonderful visit. However, our time together makes me fully aware that I have passed out of the stage of ever wanting to have any more kids. We sit together and chat, and I can't help but feel so blessed that I'm not pregnant or a new mom. This broken neck sure is a ton easier than those two roles.

July 14, 2017

Oh my, I'm tired! Either this healing business is legitimately draining me, or maybe it's the heat and humidity. All week, I've been heading to bed early, feeling beaten and exhausted. It's not that I can't do what I want to do, it's that I can barely even stay awake.

Still, there are activities on the calendar and work to be done. This morning, my mother-in-law came over and took us on a pre-school field trip. I had committed to this event about a month ago. I wasn't sure how it would go with my broken neck and a bunch of preschoolers, but it went well. We all enjoyed our time in the museum and with each other. My boys sure do love to spend time with their grandparents.

My oldest son's former preschool teacher has a sister-in-law who's an ER nurse. When she found out that I was in an accident, she asked her sister-in-law if she was working then. It turns out that I was the talk of the ER.

Her sister-in-law had not been working, but she knew all about how I seemed pretty fine when I came in and then, bam!, I was diagnosed with a broken neck. For some odd reason, I felt very proud that I could be an ER legend for a day. It kind of made me feel like I just won a contest. "Luckiest Gal in the World" is what my sash would say. My tiara would be small and delicate so it could be strategically placed to miss the road rash on my scalp, and it would be safely secured so it couldn't fall and touch my busted eyebrow.

When we were about done talking, my son's former teacher leaned in. "I just have to ask. Did you make it home?"

"Yes, I made it home face-first, but I was safe. He didn't tag me out."

"I'm sorry. I just had to ask."

"I know. You're not the only one. It was a pretty important detail for the ER staff, too."

After the field trip, we took the boys to the sitter, and I went to work. When I write for my blog, I write posts on how to do different yoga poses and Pilates exercises. Videos accompany those posts.

Today, my yoga teacher and mentor, Stephanie, volunteered to come over and film some how-to videos on various yoga poses. I asked her to teach some spinal extension and spinal rotation poses because I won't be doing those for a while.

I enjoyed having her over to film, and I think I'll ask her to help me out with poses even in the future when I'm not injured. It was interesting to film the videos and show the interaction between us. Plus, when we discuss why and how we do different poses, it might bring some depth to my content.

This afternoon, my friend Katie came over to drive me to pick up the boys. I was relieved when she said that she, too, was exhausted. For the record, she has no major breaks or injuries from which she is recovering—maybe it is our stifling weather.

Summertime Blues

5

July 15, 2017

Oh, how I wanted pizza for lunch. I placed our order, and the boys and I began our wait. We decided that when the pizza came, we would draw the shades, watch *Home Alone*, and pretend it was winter. It was awesome! Such a great use of a Saturday afternoon. After the movie, the three of us took a very long, glorious nap.

Then, after our nap, Katie came over again to drive us to my friend Susanne's 40th birthday party. This was my first real outing—a social event where acquaintances would ask questions. Mostly, people were concerned about how I was feeling. When I told them I felt fine, they seemed to doubt my answer, asking, "Isn't that neck brace uncomfortable?"

In fact, I wish they would have not asked that follow-up questions. I wish they would have said they were glad I was okay and feeling fine, glad I hadn't been injured worse, or something along those lines. However, that rarely happened.

"You must be so uncomfortable."

It was a statement, an insistence almost. And, although I was uncomfortable, I didn't want to talk about it. I was afraid that if I started talking about how I uncomfortable I was, I would be perceived as being ungrateful or unappreciative for the relatively little damage that I incurred.

I was uncomfortable for so many reasons:

1. I was physically uncomfortable from my injuries, the heat, and my plastic neck brace.
2. Whenever people looked at me, their faces revealed the shock and horror that they felt.
3. They would often come talk to me. Of course, they had to tell me how lucky I was to be alive, that people die from broken necks all the time, and that I could have died right there in front of my kids.

Why do people do that? Do they actually think I don't realize how close to death I was? It was nothing I hadn't already thought myself but having to talk to acquaintances about it *all evening long* was tiresome.

The reason I was most uncomfortable, though, was that I was happy to have my neck brace. Everyone was expecting me to wish I didn't have it or something along those lines, but I was glad to have it. That piece of plastic is what is keeping me from needing surgery, being paralyzed, or even being dead.

I love the neck brace for all that it is doing for me. Frankly, I'm petrified of the idea of spending time without it. Although I look forward to having the doctor tell me that my facet joint has healed, I do not look forward to ditching my plastic safety blanket and rejoining the rest of the folks who don't walk around with neck protection 24/7.

July 16, 2017

You know, some days are much harder than others. Boy, oh, boy, it was hard to make time to go to my computer. When afternoon naptime rolled around, I was desperate for a break, and I think I slept over two hours.

Of course, this can lead to issues for sleeping at night. The two-year-old was having a rough time going to sleep. I was listening for every little noise, convinced that it was the tiny munchkin on his way to wake me. He never did.

Instead, three times my very enthusiastic and loud cat brought me his toy. Don't get me wrong, I'm thankful that my cat brings me toys instead of birds, rabbits, or mice. However, he likes to bring me presents as I'm about to fall asleep.

I am almost sleeping and then, "YOWL! RUH RUH RAHHH!" Before owning this cat, I have never heard a noise like it. However, once he started making this noise, the other cats started doing their best imitation of it.

You see, when the cat's mouth is open, it produces a lovelier, louder tone. This toy provides an appropriate space in his mouth so that he can make a maximal yowl. It's a truly remarkable noise, especially in the darkness of night when I'm trying to fall asleep.

What is also funny is that he won't stop yowling until I verbally acknowledge my present and tell him that it's time for bed. Sometimes, I have to be insistent and pat the bed for him to join me. He rarely joins me, but he does quit yowling.

Today, I'm pretty jealous of other people's normal summers. This is petty and small, I know. Truly, I am elated simply to be alive—not to mention the fact that I have no muscle weakness or nerve damage. Let me be clear, I'm most thankful for where I am.

If I didn't get that dumb idea to have our bases go up, then downhill, I would be packing for a two-week camping trip. We were supposed to travel across the country and make our way ultimately to Orlando. First, though, we were going to spend some days in Savannah, Georgia, my top bucket-list destination. Then, we would travel down the Atlantic side of Florida. I would also get to see Daytona, another location on my bucket list, before we would go hang out at Cape Canaveral. Finally, after enjoying the beach and Space Center, we would make our way over for a week of fun in Orlando. Since the kids are still pretty young, I envisioned a mix of Disney and fun at the pool.

However, a neck brace changes all that. Instead, we're going for a weeklong vacation at my folks' house. They live near St. Louis, and we'll have plenty to do and lots of fun. Still, I'm a little disappointed that I'm not going to have my dream vacation.

It seems like every time I go on Facebook, someone is posting pictures from their vacation. Oh, Colorado! Oh, Gulf Shores! And I'm over here staying inside my house because it's too freaking hot for me to go outside, losing any sort of tan that I had, and killing time until September.

This is not the type of person I am. I'm never killing time, waiting for one phase to pass so I can get to the next one. I try to do what I can to appreciate and celebrate life, but some days are a little harder than others.

Offering My Hard-Earned Advice

6

How to Wear a Cervical Collar Comfortably

The doctor has informed you that for a while, you will be wearing foamy plastic that is Velcroed around your neck. You're thankful that you're not dead or paralyzed but are still apprehensive about your comfort level in your future days.

Fear not! I have some tips to help keep you comfortable during this essential healing time.

1. *Always* follow your doctor's orders precisely.
2. If there is some instinct within you that tells you that you should not follow your doctor's orders precisely, get a second opinion with another doctor. You are ultimately the one responsible for making choices about your body so if something feels wrong, seek help from another medical professional.
3. Your neck brace is probably adjustable, at least, the model I have is. It would stand to reason that since neck lengths vary, neck braces should be adjustable. For my brace, my doctor told me that I should feel like my jaw and chin rest comfortably on my brace. Then, you want to get it tight enough to be supportive, but keep it loose enough that you don't choke yourself.

4. If you only read one tip, this is the one: *Relax your shoulders!* Maybe you think that this is an odd tip, but science supports me. Your neck is a certain length. Presumably, you have followed tip #3 and adjusted your neck brace to fit you correctly. Your neck and neck brace are both a constant measurement; they will never change lengths.

   If you start to get tense, and your shoulders start to slide up toward your ears, you end up applying an unwanted traction to the cervical spine. Since your cervical spine is the area you want to immobilize, the area with the injury, you *do not want to apply force.* Any time your shoulders raise, your neck brace will shift upward and push your head upward, too. Therefore, keep your shoulders relaxed at all times.

5. Use your pillow wisely. Obviously, sleeping on your back is going to be your best bet. If you are flat on your back, try to use a very thin pillow. I have found that if I get myself placed so that my shoulders are right at the bottom edge of the pillow, I feel comfortable. If my shoulders are on the pillow at all, the lift makes me strain and feel uncomfortable. Also, bravely I discovered that I can fold my pillow in half to make an appropriate prop for me to sleep on my side. This leads me to my next point.

6. Do whatever you need to do to enable you to sleep comfortably. For days, I exclusively slept on my back, and sometimes my legs were out straight, sometimes they were bent. Finally, I reached the point where my low back started tightening up. In the middle of the night, I would have to sit up and lean forward, giving my low back a break.

Find several comfortable sleeping positions. If you need pillows to help you get placed, make sure to set up your pillows before you fall asleep. You want to minimize the work you have to do to make yourself comfortable in the middle of the night.

7. Be smart when you get out of bed.

- When you first wake up, let yourself wake up fully. It would be a real pity if you hurt yourself because you were half asleep and not paying attention.
- When you're awake, recruit your abs to help; then move.
- Roll onto your side closest to the edge of the bed.
- Use your arms to push yourself up to a seated position. However, if you think that would put too much strain on your neck or if your arms are lacking in strength or sensation, recruit your abs, and sit straight up.

8. Literally, before you make any movement, recruit your abs. Want to stand after sitting? Recruit your abs. Want to take a walk? Recruit your abs. Want to lie down in bed? Recruit your abs.

9. Imagine what perfect posture would look like; then, try to keep your body in that position for as long as possible.

10. Take breaks and rest flat on your back.

July 19, 2017

10 Things to Avoid While Living with a Neck Brace

After living with a neck brace for a few weeks, I've discovered there are some important things to avoid while letting a broken neck heal. I'm doing things that I hope will improve my recovery—

more calcium, less soda, continuous collar wearing, and mindful movement.

Here are some observations about what to avoid while wearing my least-favorite accessory. I created this list because I wish that my doctor's office would have had something like this for me when I left the first day—something to tell me what to do and what to avoid. I sure would have rather read about *what not to do*—than experienced it. Please let my pain be your gain, and learn from my mistakes.

1. Obviously, any activities that your doctor has advised you to cease, you should stop.

2. Don't do anything that could jar your spine. No roller coasters, horseback riding, roller skating, bike riding, and *no running*.

3. Don't lift anything above the weight set by your doctor. For me, it's 10 pounds. If I'm not supposed to lift anything greater than 10 pounds, it also stands to reason that I should not push or pull anything greater than 10 pounds.

4. Limit reaching your arms overhead. Many of the nerves for our arms come from our cervical spine. Some of the muscles that control movement of your scapulas (shoulder blades) are located right below your cervical spine. Therefore, it's best to reach overhead only if absolutely necessary. For some people, this advice may be moot because pain from a damaged nerve in your neck may prohibit you from lifting your arms overhead.

5. Do not rotate your spine. With your cervical area stabilized, the rest of your spine is now more vulnerable to injury. Yes, some rotation from the rest of your spine is fine. However, you should avoid large twists as well as bending

straight to the side. A big bend to the side is a great way to quickly mess up your low back.

6. When you need to pick up something, don't hinge from the hips exclusively. You also want to bend deeply at your knees. Keep your spine as straight as you can while you lift. As always, engage your abs before doing anything.

7. Don't let your head get lower than your chest and hips. Yes, I learned this lesson myself. When the head is lower than the chest or hips, that is a natural form of traction. In this case, traction is applied to the neck with help from gravity. Gravity gently tugs on your neck and head to help create space and relieve compression among the cervical vertebrae. This is a wonderful thing, except for when you're trying to stabilize your cervical spine to allow it to heal from an injury.

8. Avoid stress and tension. It's fair to say that you have enough on your plate. Do your best to avoid additional stress. If you feel yourself getting tense, take a break and lie down and meditate. Lie down on your back to combat the effects of gravity, and practice deep breathing to help you relax. Plus, if your shoulders start lifting toward your ears, it will apply pressure on your neck brace. Your neck brace then applies pressure to your jawline and, once again, you have a form of traction for your neck.

9. Don't let your body get stiff and tight. I know, this one sounds like a contradiction since, if you're like me, you're only allowed to walk. However, do your best to stretch yourself out. For me, this means sitting with my legs straight in front of me in Staff pose (Dandasana), getting into the hip-opening position for Bound angle pose (Baddha Konasana), and maybe even sitting in Hero pose

(Virasana). (Directions to practice these basic yoga poses are found on pages 164, 167, and 169 respectively.)

Oddly, I find that my biceps also need a good stretch. In the middle of the night, my tight shoulders want me to bend my elbows and rest my palms on my stomach. I'd guess that I do this for a good portion of my sleep. Then, in the morning, I'm starting to feel like I have short, stubby arms like a T-Rex.

Don't lose focus on your goal. Healing a break in a bone takes quite a bit of time and effort. Be patient with the process. In the scheme of your life, God willing, this time will be a drop in the bucket. *Make your number one goal every day be to heal your break, and do whatever is in your power that day to reach your goal.*

July 20, 2017

It's our 15th anniversary, and my husband is working. Plus, it's extremely hot, and my crazy kids want to play outside. I've already had to threaten an early bedtime, which made them quit fighting and start playing together, but, I'm going to be honest, I'm not sure how much longer I'm going to last. It's 6:39 p.m.

At different points last night, I woke up with eyebrow pain. Earlier yesterday, I played with raising my eyebrows. I wanted to make sure the muscles in that area were all working. When I lifted my eyebrow, it ended up being quite painful, and I had a dull throb of pain the rest of the day.

I know that this will stop sometime, but feeling a sharp pain above your eye in the middle of the night is bothersome. What throws me is that it appears to be a pain generated by the air from my ceiling fan. Nothing makes me feel more like the "Princess and the Pea" than the notion of having intense pain from the gentle breeze generated by my ceiling fan. How pathetic!

It's another hair-washing night, so I'm grumpy about that, too. I don't think I've said anything yet but, aside from the anxiety that I feel when I take off my collar and shower, the hair-washing showers are a little painful. It feels like I'm losing the strength in my neck muscles (I am) so, after about 10 minutes, my neck starts to get tired.

Maybe you're thinking that 10 minutes is plenty of time to shower. Well, with a cervical spine injury, it's not. To make sure that I don't mess up my neck, I avoid doing lots of activities with my arms above shoulder level. Guess where my shampoo is. It's in line with my forehead. My conditioner is even higher. Suffice to say, if I don't have everything planned and then work according to plan, I can get tired and sore very quickly.

Plus, my eyebrow is already hurting and my neck is starting to get sore—either from the stress of my crazy kids or from sitting at the computer writing. Damn. Both are equally likely.

I think I'm going to make myself some chocolate milk and find a nice, mindless game show to watch on TV, or maybe I'll watch an old episode of *Cheers*.

July 21, 2017

I decided to kind of rest today. I worked first thing this morning with some clients, had my husband take me to the bank, then I watched *Big Brother* on TV. I took a nap and hit snooze more times than I had planned. Then, even though I wasn't very motivated to write, I wrote a blog post I was happy with, edited it, and scheduled it.

Our friends Doug and Amy are visiting, and it has been about two or three years since the last time. Man, *it's like soup for your soul to see old friends*.

July 22, 2017

I worked this morning; then, my husband went to work. The kids and I needed to have a little time for a nap before my mother-in-law picked us up to take us to my nephew's birthday party. When I said that we were going up to take a nap, my two-year-old said, "Nap!" and ran upstairs. By the time I arrived, he was totally naked and jumping on my older son's bed. He had peed in his potty, dumped it in the big potty, and, I guess, was doing some victory bouncing. It made my day.

The nap was very short, probably only about 20 minutes. The little one is used to getting about two and a half hours in the afternoon. When we came home from the party, I popped in a movie, and we watched it on the couch. The two-year-old fell asleep on me around 6:45 and slept all the way through the night. Even when I made dinner, he slept. With lights blazing, he slept. The kid was tired.

July 23, 2017

We woke this morning to some sad news. Something killed two of our chickens. My husband thinks we have a raccoon or possum getting into the chicken coop and attacking the girls. I have always been very protective of the chickens. It's not odd for me to chase off hawks and corral the girls to safety within their coop. With this heat, I'm not outside as much as I would be normally, so I can't offer much protection.

This neck brace is hot. It's like wearing a wool scarf wrapped tightly around your neck at all times. There's this cutout on the front, but I don't know whom they think they're fooling. This collar is still its own sauna, but that's okay. It's a legitimate reason to stay inside and enjoy the air conditioning.

We had a huge storm and my husband was called into work. As a lineman, this means that he will work 16-hour days until everyone's power is restored. Normally, this isn't too big of a deal for the boys and me. We miss him and try to deliver snacks to him if he's working around our area. However, with this neck brace, our status-quo storm operations are non-existent.

That's a big reason why I want to get my collar off. When my husband gets called into work, I feel like I'm in a scramble to get organized to get drivers to help me run the boys and do other essential errands. Thank goodness we have such great family and friends here. I would be at a loss if we lived in a town where we didn't have such a great support system.

Taking Care of Your Personal Hygiene

7

July 24, 2017

Taking a Shower

It has been a real learning curve, figuring out how to shower safely. First, make sure to give yourself double the amount of time you would require to shower uninjured. You want to make sure you won't end up rushing to get done. Rushing can cause us to do something that our bodies may later regret.

Next, make sure you do not tilt your head back into the water—it would be a huge mistake. Pick a spot straight in front of you to focus on, and try to keep your head level throughout the shower.

Get your showerhead adjusted so a good deal of water is coming down straight on the top of your head. If the water hits you on the back of the head, it won't feel as good. The water pressure is a force you have to resist to maintain neutral. When the water hits you right on the top of your head, your spine doesn't have to work to stay in neutral. This adjustment will allow you to get wet but not be in pain.

Your next step is to clean yourself. If you can, grab hold of something secured to your shower. I keep a hand on the tracking bar of our adjustable showerhead. This way, if I slip, I have something stable that I can grab. Maybe you would feel safer by sitting on the shower floor. Do what you have to. No one is judging you.

Follow these easy steps to wash yourself:
- Take your time.
- Take breaks if needed.
- Keep your head still at all times.
- Don't forget to clean the back of your neck.
- Dry yourself and get your neck brace back on. If you're like me, the brace brings comfort.

Drying Your Hair

If you have mid-length to long hair, you have an additional challenge—managing long, wet hair. I have yet to figure out how the heck I'm supposed to towel dry my hair without lowering my head. You might remember from reading (or personal experience), it's a terrible idea to let your head be lower than your heart because of the traction on your neck. However, I have yet to find a good way to towel dry my hair that doesn't involve me lowering my head. Just rubbing my towel on my upright head doesn't seem to get the job done well.

Or, there's the possibility that you may want to skip towel drying and move straight to the hair dryer. This, of course, would involve you holding something at shoulder level, which might not even be possible if you have nerve damage or muscle weakness. Then, you have to hold and move the hair dryer for an even longer time because your hair is sopping wet.

My very least favorite part of the long, wet hair/neck brace scenario is that once you're done, you're going to discover that the shorter hairs have all slicked down against your neck and tucked themselves inside your neck brace. Thus, you have damp hair stuck firmly to your neck and held in place by a now-soggy neck brace pad.

July 25, 2017

Today, I woke up with menstrual cramps. I knew the day would come when I would have my period while wearing this neck brace, but I have been dreading it. However, the cramps were an unpleasant surprise.

It's very frustrating to think of all the things I could do to help myself but constantly have to tell myself "No" because I'm not cleared to exercise. I can't do any yoga or Pilates, which, incidentally, help a great deal with pain management for menstrual cramps. Instead, I have to go around with this gut bloat and low back pain.

Parents and Helpful Friends

8

Today Mom calls and asks if I want to go visit my grandma while I'm out there on vacation. I don't even know if I can handle the long car ride to my parents' house, let alone the additional car time that it would take to get to Grammy's. The thought of having to make this decision right now without knowing how I'll do on a long car ride makes my head spin.

*****

One of my very good friends, someone who has brought me food and given me rides, was admitted to the hospital to have emergency back surgery. She has rheumatoid arthritis (RA) and fibromyalgia, and the first half of this year has been terrible for her. She had completed physical therapy for back surgery, been cleared for a few weeks, but then innocently picked up a package and lost feeling in several key areas in her pelvis. I'm sick about it.

I'm upset that she has these shitty diseases that constantly attack her and make her vulnerable to injury. I'm upset that the doctor couldn't do the spinal fusion that she needed initially because insurance wouldn't cover it if she didn't have this other, lesser procedure done first. I'm upset that because I have this annoying neck brace, I can't do anything to help out their family as one of my best friends goes into the hospital for the fourth or fifth time this year.

From her hospital bed, my friend called me to tell me that she couldn't help drive me on Friday like we had originally planned. She said would send her husband to drive the shift. Can you believe that? I said, "Uh. No. I can handle this. It's more important that he helps you and your family. I'll ask someone else."

I found a replacement for the Friday driving shift. Then, I received a message from one of my Thursday rides saying she couldn't help out either.

After I got that covered, my ride who volunteered to drive to and from preschool asks if she can beg out. Of course I have no problem with that, but I am getting very stressed out trying to get these shifts covered, wrap up swimming lessons, wrap up preschool, get ready for vacation, journal every day, and get all my articles done for my website before we go on vacation so I don't want to have to work the entire time we're gone. I am totally stressed out with all this scheduling.

Jeez! Now that I've done all my venting, I want to brag on my kids. We went to swimming class for my five-year-old's last lesson tonight. To my surprise, the two-year-old wanted to get into his swim diaper and floaty. I thought he'd play on the steps, but he jumped in and swam right after my older son and the teacher. He wanted to be part of the lesson and do everything that his big brother was doing.

Both boys did a fantastic job. The older one was going underwater all the time like he was a fish, and the younger one had some moments where he tipped on his side but he stayed calm. It was such a joy to watch the boys swim. Much appreciation to my gal pal, Jenna, who did the monster trek of picking the older one up from preschool, going to swim lessons with us, and taking us out for chocolate shakes afterwards.

This is the absolute, 100 percent truth: Without my friends and our family, we would be lost, and I would be losing my mind.

Tips for a Good Night's Sleep with a Broken Neck

9

July 26, 2017

In the time that I've been healing from my injury, I have made several observations about changes I can make to positively impact my comfort, health, and happiness. In particular, I have tried to master sleeping well with a broken neck.

Many people normally have difficulties sleeping. Frequently, I have people concerned about whether I can sleep with my neck brace. Yes, I had a steep learning curve, but I feel like I've mastered it.

Additionally, I've tried to make my tips universal—you don't *have* to have a broken neck to benefit from these tips about sleeping well.

1. Relax your shoulders away from your ears. As your shoulders tense, they will push against the neck brace. This will push against your jaw and create a mild traction for your cervical spine. *This will hurt*.

    As you feel your shoulders tense and rise toward your ears, slide them down. Rock side-to-side to get your shoulder blades in the correct neutral position on your back. When your shoulder blades are slightly pinned on your back, they will be less likely to rise and become a problem.

2. Plan for comfortable sleeping on your back. Doctors say that it's best for people to sleep on their backs. With a broken neck, back sleeping is definitely your best option. Because most of the time you will be sleeping on your back, come up with some ideas of ways you can change positions but still be on your back.

   For example, you might work on bending one or both knees. Right after I broke my neck, this is what I would do. I was so tired that my feet stayed firmly anchored while I slept. My bent knees were enough of a change that my body could easily sleep this way. You might also think of possibly using pillows as props. For me, because pillows tend to be an obstacle, I didn't go this route.

3. Make sure you have the correct pillow for your sleeping style. If you are stable enough that you think you could sleep on your side, make sure you have a pillow plan. For example, back sleepers need a very thin pillow. With this sleep style, you're looking for something to support your cervical curve in your neck. For side sleepers, though, you need quite a bit more pillow.

   To determine how thick your pillow needs to be, roll completely onto your side. Make sure that you are stacked right on top of your shoulder joint. (The tendency is for the shoulder capsule to be slightly in front of the body, which causes misalignment.) Even though your body weight is squarely on your shoulder, you should still be very comfortable and able to move your arm with ease. Keep your head lifted to neutral. Ideally, the space between your mattress and ear should be filled with appropriately supportive pillow. Just in case you're wondering, you should not at all attempt to sleep on your stomach.

4. Manage your pain meds. Using pain meds while sleeping can be a double-edged sword. On the one hand, you don't want to wake up in the middle of the night with pain. On the other hand, pain medications can cause you to be drowsy during the day.

   This may result in long naps, which could prevent you from getting a good, restful night's sleep. I was feeling sluggish during the day and having difficulty sleeping at night, so I quit taking my acetaminophen. It was the correct decision. My head cleared, I was productive during the day, and I slept like a champ at night.

5. When you lay down to sleep at night, focus on your task. You are going to sleep. This is going to help your mind rest and your body heal. One of the most important things you will do for yourself is sleep. If your mind is racing, focus on the task at hand—you are repairing any damage your day may have done to your body.

20 Reasons Why I Love My Neck Brace

10

Without our sense of humor, we are nothing.
– Sarah Stockett

I'm sure someone important said that once. Maybe they said something just like that but not in those exact words. Or, maybe I'm the famous person who said that. Yes, I'm the famous person who said that.

Frequently, when I am stressed, I use my sense of humor as a coping mechanism. Although my healing process has gone very well and I have been blessed to be relatively pain-free, it is still a bummer to wear this neck brace throughout the summer.

It's hot, I can't swim with my kids, I can't turn my head, and I live with a constant fear that I will do something stupid and end up paralyzing myself or accidentally dying. This is all just a little too much drama for me, especially in the summertime.

So, to escape all this drama, I created these humorous 20 Reasons Why I Love My Neck Brace.

1. That beautiful neutral posture I've always wanted? Check.
2. Finally! A force stronger than my shoulders to beat them down away from my ears.
3. Napping through car rides is a breeze.

4. Because I am no longer able to work and eat at the same time, I've been watching more TV. *Stranger Things* is amazing!

5. Having to use your non-dominant hand to put on eye makeup kind of leaves you like a walking work of art. *Is that a Picasso?*

6. I look like a rock star when I play my ukulele because I can't look at the strings.

7. My double chin vanished!

8. The back of my neck brace cradles my skull like a Disney villain dress collar. I'm thinking of wearing a skull cap to accentuate the look.

9. No one expects anything from you anymore. Waking up and putting on clothes are your only obligations.

10. Let it be known that July 1, I got to watch whatever I wanted to watch on TV whenever I wanted to watch it. And all I had to do was break my neck.

11. I don't have to change the cat box. This is the first long stretch of time since 2011 that I haven't had to change the cat box.

12. I don't have to wonder if I should go for a walk. Hell no! It's too hot for that!

13. It's possibly less noticeable when I roll my eyes. Maybe.

14. Everyone is so polite.

15. Finally, I have an excuse for why I need 10-12 hours of sleep.

16. I don't have to worry about plucking chin or neck hairs. If I can't see them, no one else can either.

17. The comparison of me being dead or paralyzed often results in "Oh, you look so good" compliments, and I'll take them. Gladly.

18. When eating in public, the neck brace gives me a good reason to tuck my napkin in under my chin and save the front of my shirt from my sloppy eating.
19. Ice cream? I think so. I need all the calcium I can get. I'm healing bones here, people!
20. I'm totally going to incorporate the neck brace in my Halloween costume this year.

Out and About

11

July 27, 2017

I have still been having pain and discomfort with my eyebrow wound. Last night, we had a storm rolling in and my face hurt as badly as when it first split open. I had a soda with dinner, and it helped me feel better. I'm not sure what it is, but there's something about soda that helps ease my storm-related headaches.

Today, I decided to try moving my eyebrow again. This still ended up being quite painful, and even when I wasn't doing anything with my eyebrow, I felt a dull throb of pain.

Last night, I thought this lump over my eyebrow might be some sort of cyst. I took a grapefruit seed extract capsule and decided to take a garlic capsule for good measure. When I woke up this morning, I couldn't believe it. My cyst-like bump was noticeably smaller. I decided to take garlic and grapefruit seed extract today as well. The idea that maybe I can get this thing to go away excites me.

July 28, 2017

I'm taking the day off. I worked with clients this morning then took a walk. Walking by myself scared me. I'm obviously an easy target, and some very seedy people moved into the neighborhood recently. To up the odds for my personal safety, I opted to walk at noon in full sunlight, even though it was extremely hot.

As I reached the house where the seedy people have been living, I came upon the homeowner. Talking to him, I learned that he had been renting out the top part of his house to help him cover rent. After a visit from the drug strike force, a couple of visits from the police, and the realization that the upstairs of his house was involved in drug-related activity, thankfully he served eviction notices to all.

Now, I feel a lot better about walking on my own. It seems more likely that I will be able to stroll in peace and not have to wonder who's coming up behind me. I still don't think I'll push my luck and go walking with the kids.

Also, while walking, a couple of small cramps appeared in my upper trapezius. In case you don't know anatomy, the upper trapezius is the muscle that runs from your neck out to the tip of your shoulder. When people rub their necks, they often rub this muscle. It's notorious for causing neck pain because of its origin, which is right along the vertebrae of your neck.

The cramp wasn't terrible; it relaxed right away. However, I can't wait to get my neck brace off so I can get a good massage. It will be nice to have somebody rub these muscles.

After my walk, I started binge-watching *Stranger Things* on TV. This show has caused my productivity to significantly decrease. Even when I was in an acetaminophen and pain-related stupor, even when I was hanging out with my folks, I was still more productive than I am right now.

This show is wonderful. Great writing, mystery, suspense, drama, the 1980s—it has it all. I fully intend to write something tomorrow but, if I don't, it will be because I'm watching *Stranger Things*.

July 29, 2017

I am thankful for every workday that my husband gets time to come home and cook dinner. Tonight, he fixed brats. You might think this is crazy, but I have no idea how to cook brats. I know that this is within my grasp; it's something I can learn. However, I haven't.

I tried. I cooked the brats once, and they were slimy and nasty. I think this is because I have no grill skills. Maybe I should work on that.

A Month After the Accident and My St. Louis Vacation

12

July 30, 2017

Today, we headed out to my parents' house for vacation, almost a five-hour car ride away. I won't lie—it was kind of painful. I thought it would be no big deal to take a nap with the neck brace, but that didn't prove to be true.

Honestly, sitting straight up was the most comfortable position. It hurt when I slightly reclined my seat, and I developed this pain on the back of my head. Maybe it was my hair tie or maybe the plastic of my neck brace was hitting me in a bad spot, but it *was not* comfortable.

This vacation is a whole crapshoot. We certainly run the risk that I won't feel well and end up sleeping the whole week at my parents' house, which wouldn't be that bad, I guess.

Dad and I went for a walk after dinner. The temperature was perfect, and I didn't get too sweaty. We ran into someone I went to school with who I haven't seen for years. We were friends in elementary school and then went our separate ways. I couldn't even remember the last time I saw her.

Yet, as Dad and I walked toward her, I knew exactly who she was. I would know her anywhere, but particularly standing in front of her dad's house, the house we played at as kids. As we approached, I couldn't help but feel like I was in some sort of odd time warp, like I was back in the fourth grade when we first met. I'm not sure why, but the whole situation felt energizing, almost magical. Nothing profound was said. There was nothing that should really indicate that this moment was spectacular (or even particularly memorable), but I can feel it. I feel like something wonderful has just happened, and I can't wait to discover what the Universe has in store for me next.

July 31, 2017

Our family visited the Transportation Museum, ate lunch with my aunt and uncle, and looked at Airstream campers. I felt great while I was doing all of those things. When we returned to my parents' the house, I took a nap. I thought I'd make it a quick one, which would allow me to watch some *Stranger Things* or write.

Neither of those could entice me out of bed. I napped until almost 6 p.m., and I think I could have slept longer. I'm not sure if it's the activity, heat, or the healing process; but I certainly would like to have my regular energy levels back.

When I finally woke up, my husband and I went for a walk. Tonight was much more humid. I felt muscles in my neck twitch, and getting sweaty made me feel extremely uncomfortable. However, when we went out for ice cream later, the temperature was perfect.

After my shower, I decided to change my neck brace pads. I've been active in the past week, and the pads are getting a little nasty. This scares me. I'm worried that something won't be the correct place, and I'll accidentally mess up my healing process. Or, maybe I won't get things right, and I'll be uncomfortable when I go to sleep tonight. I hope not because I'm still tired—and I'm hoping that I sleep like a champ.

August 1, 2017

All of us drove up to Decatur, Illinois to visit my grandma. We took two separate vehicles and caravanned into town. Sometimes one of us would have to stop for a bathroom break or food, so we would call the other car. As someone who can easily remember the days when phones were firmly attached to house walls, I have to say that I love the conveniences that come with technology. Being able to call my parents made the car trip so much easier than it would have been otherwise.

The ride was quite uninteresting, and I was relieved because I wasn't too sure how my beaten-up body would handle another car trip. Thankfully, our drive from St. Louis was about two and a half hours. When we popped in a movie for the boys in the backseat, time seemed to go faster.

After we checked into the hotel, we caravanned over to pick up my grandma for dinner. She's 92 and still living on her own in her apartment.

During dinner, she kept asking me if my neck hurts much. I'm not sure if that's a reflection on the way I look or her bad memory. Boy, I hope it's more of a reflection on her bad memory. I don't want to be walking around looking half-dead.

After dinner, we went back to the hotel where my husband and boys went swimming. The pool was small, but the boys had a great time because we were the only ones there. The two-year-old was fearless and almost hit his head on the wall two or three times.

I hope we don't have to take him to the hospital while I still have my neck brace. Gosh, our family would look like a mess then.

August 2, 2017

Our stay in Decatur was brief. We came back to St. Louis today. It was nice to have visited my grandma. I hope that she is doing well, but I couldn't tell. She has this habit of not wearing her hearing aids, which makes having a true, genuine conversation difficult. Still, if we can't hold a deep conversation, I can tell that she loves me and that she cares.

When we all arrived back in St. Louis, we ate at this wonderful restaurant near my parents' house. Back in 2002, my husband and I had our wedding rehearsal dinner there. My folks beat us there and found a table. We were past the lunch rush and well before the dinner crowd, so the restaurant patrons had thinned out.

As we walked in, I thought I caught a glimpse of a guy with whom I used to go to elementary school. We sat down with my parents, and it turned out he was our waiter. I couldn't believe it. Here was my friend Tom, who I hadn't seen in almost 20 years, and I knew him immediately.

It made my heart so happy to see him. All of the good memories about our time together—including a funny thing that he told me back in sixth grade—came flooding back, filling me with happiness and warmth.

We started talking about others we went to elementary school with, and then I asked him when his high school reunion was. He said, "Oh, I probably won't go. I already keep in touch with everyone I want to talk to."

I couldn't believe it! My husband had said almost the same thing verbatim a few weeks earlier. That's when I made the connection; Tom is a lot like my husband. All this time, I had loved Tom's laid back nature and easy-going sense of humor. Tom is one of those guys that I would think, *Man, I'd love for my husband to meet him someday. They'd get along really well.* Now, it was happening.

When we finished lunch, I had an email saying our local university is looking for a yoga instructor. Years ago, I filled in for a colleague and taught a semester of Pilates and Cardio Dance. I'm thinking this may be a good opportunity for me—if my neck brace is off in time.

August 3, 2017

It's Thursday of vacation week. After a delayed start, we made our way to the City Museum. We played inside before gathering and heading up to the roof. The boys walked across the steppingstones in the water, then we headed for the Ferris wheel, which only Dad and I decided to ride.

Almost immediately, this woman behind me asks, "Excuse me, is your name Sarah?"

At first, I was confused. Surely, she wasn't talking to me. I turned around and it was my high school ex-boyfriend's sister, Amy, who I always liked. She caught me up about her family. It's funny how quickly you can describe the past 20 years while you the wait for a Ferris wheel.

I can't help but wonder: *What is the universe trying to tell me?* Three people from my past, three people that I *enjoyed*, appear in front of me. Mind you, since I can't turn my head, my observation skills are not what they were. These people have to literally be right in front of my face in order for me to see them. What do their appearances mean?

On top of all these fortunate surprise connections, I'm feeling very good. My neck is feeling fine. My eyebrow scar continues to persist, but I have less pain. However, the scar is quite sensitive to cold air blowing on it—which feels like a person with sensitive teeth eating ice cream because it goes right to the bone.

I have to say, though, my left thigh is kind of troubling me. It looks fine enough, but when the light shines on it just right, you can still see the outline of the bruise. Plus, there is a noticeable divot on my leg where it hit the step. This is a permanent edema that looks like I've had my thigh pressed against a bar of sorts, except I haven't. I'm hoping I can use The Orb massage ball to break up the adhesion and repair my dent.

*****

Last night, I thought about whether or not I should apply for the teaching job at the university. I decided that I should. I think that I would have fun and that I have a lot of information to share with new students. Also, I think I could structure the class so that it would be a nice mix of education and yoga practice. I'm going to send an email first thing in the morning.

But first, my husband and I are going out on a date night. My folks are watching the kids, so we picked a nice sushi place. Where I come from, our grocery store is our nice sushi place. Also, our brother-in-law does a pretty good job making California rolls.

We took our time eating and decided to check out the movie theater. Nothing we wanted to see was playing, so we decided to go shopping to buy my folks a new coffeemaker. Then, we went to a big bookstore because we don't have a bookstore in town anymore.

Like a couple of people with no responsibilities, we wandered the aisles. I settled in the children's section and read Mo Willems' books. My husband looked for loftier entertainment and ended up with a book on writing. Since his freshman comp class last semester, he has become increasingly interested in writing and the rules of the English language. This book suits me perfectly.

August 4, 2017

In Missouri, we have a tax-free weekend for back-to-school shopping. It's normally the first weekend of August. Since tax-free weekend coincided with our vacation, all of us went shopping.

Bargain shopping is a particularly wonderful activity for my mom and me. For my dad and husband, it is brutally punishing. Mom and I did our best to respect their lack of enthusiasm as she pushed my sons in a cart through the store, allowing them to choose any clothes or school necessities that they wanted.

Later that night, we all had dinner in a nice restaurant with one of my best friends, Erin. We have been best friends since seventh grade. As adults, we don't spend nearly enough time talking with each other or hanging out. When we do get together, it's like a day hasn't passed since I've seen her last.

After dinner, I rode back to my parents' house with Erin so we could catch up on all the things that you might want to tell your best friend when her parents aren't around. When we returned to the house, we decided to hang out on the back patio while my dad played baseball with my boys. For hours, Erin, my husband, and I chatted about what was going on in our lives.

Erin had been on a great trip to Italy with her boyfriend. It had been a wine-influenced vacation, and it sounded exactly like some beautiful movie that I would probably watch. As she told me about the vineyards, I could practically see them. It was a perfect escape from my present condition.

But the most wonderful part about being around your best friend is that she knows when you don't want to talk about something. Unlike some acquaintances did, she never asked me if my neck hurt. In fact, aside from asking how I broke my neck, she may not have asked any more questions about it. I was so relieved.

I get so tired of talking about my neck. I'm so much more than a gal with a broken neck. However, when you wear the neck brace, it consumes you and the people around you. It becomes all that they want to talk about. You don't want to be a jerk, so you go along with their conversation. By the end of the day, though, it's emotionally draining.

August 5, 2017

Today, I had Pilates continuing education classes. Each year, I have to get continuing education credits, and I prefer to take classes with one of my original mentors, Shauna.

I was elated when I discovered that she was going to be holding a class near my parents' house while we were there on vacation. However, I knew this class would be bittersweet. Of course, I'd be so happy to see my mentor and learn new exercises. Unfortunately, I probably wouldn't be able to do anything.

My doctor had specifically said that I should not do Pilates or yoga, and I did my best to follow his orders. I was hoping that if I did everything he said, when I went for my follow-up, he would give me the good news that I could ditch my neck brace.

I went to class determined to do my best to sit still and not participate physically. It was difficult, and furthermore, I started thinking: Why shouldn't I be doing simple stretches or exercises from Pilates and yoga?

If they want me to go out walking, I would hope they would want me to stretch my legs afterward. If you don't stretch your legs after walking, the muscles in your thighs can pull on your pelvis, which can cause low back pain. The last thing I want is low back pain when I have a broken neck.

Essentially, I justified my way out of sitting still and performed only the gentlest exercises. Granted, that still meant I didn't actually do a lot in class, but it felt so good on my body. By the end of class I had decided that I needed to do more than just walk; I also needed to add in some stretches and exercises.

August 6, 2017

Vacation is over. We loaded my car and left my parents' house. Part of me hates to go, but the other part is ready to start getting everything organized so my husband and kids can go to school.

The Sex Talk

13

August 7, 2017

I t's Monday, and courtesy of his weird work schedule, my husband is still off work. Although we could technically keep the boys home with us for another day of vacation, we take them to the sitter. This allows us to work and, more importantly, have sex for the first time since I broke my neck.

Let's all take a pause here. What day is today? It's August 7th. That's a horribly long time to go without having sex. At least, for us it is.

Honestly, right after the accident, I had no sexual desires at all. I think my body was so busy healing and dealing with all the stress and trauma from the accident that it didn't have time to have any sexual impulses.

After I had healed for a while, my next obstacle was fear. I was afraid I would hurt myself while having sex, and then have to explain to doctors how exactly I got my new injury. I didn't want that to happen. When you're weighing the potential pros and cons of doing something while you have a broken neck, I think the fear of having to tell people that you've done something stupid while still in your neck brace greatly outweighs any benefit that you might get from that activity. At least, that's how it was for me.

Then, I would think about the doctor's instructions. Had he said not to have sex? No, he said no running and no horseback riding. It's the second part that gets me. Seriously, is horseback riding the #2 thing to avoid with a broken neck? Out of all the things in the world, after considering the spine-jarring activities possible, horseback riding is #2?

The more I fixate on this thought, the more I mentally compare sex to horseback riding. Then, my brain starts a little film montage of all the sexy-woman-riding-horseback scenes that I've seen through the years on TV and in film, and I start to wonder if "horseback riding" is actually code for sex.

After the brief talk with my neurosurgeon, he doesn't seem to be the kind of guy who would speak in code. I bet he would be straightforward with me. They probably aren't talking about sex.

Finally, my husband and I decided to give sex a try. I did my best to relax and focus on enjoying the moment. It felt liberating, and it was good to let my body relax and surrender to my feelings. I am so excited to add sex back into my life.

Let's Talk About Sex

In sex, even with the tamest positions, there is a certain amount of jarring to the spine when you're involved in the act. Because of this, it's important that you are absolutely certain you're ready to give it a try. Give your body time to heal from your accident. Get used to moving with your neck brace. Discover if there are any certain movements that trigger pain in your neck or other parts of your body.

Then, when you decide you're ready, focus on relaxing while you let your partner do all the hard work. Take deep breaths and focus on enjoying the present moment.

Unless, of course, your doctor has told you to avoid sexual activity. Then, you should listen to your doctor and find another way to address your sexual impulses.

August 8, 2017

Although it's Tuesday and my boys don't normally go to the sitter's today, I sent them anyway so I could get more work done. Plus, my husband is off work today, too. We're going to make some time this afternoon to have more sex. Boy, I missed being intimate—38 days is too long.

This morning, I stepped on the scale for the first time since I broke my neck. Oh, the weight gain. I've gained four pounds since the June 30 accident. I suppose it could always be worse, but four pounds in a month is not a trend I want if I'm going to wear this brace for three months. It would mean a twelve-pound overall weight gain, and I certainly don't like that number.

Still, I'm not sure what exactly to change to quit gaining weight. I'm eating a lot of dairy, but I don't think I'm eating enough to justify four extra pounds. I'll start by reducing my nightly ice cream dose. Maybe that's the cause.

An Unpleasant Surprise

14

August 9, 2017

This morning, my husband and I dropped off the boys at the sitter's and headed to the hospital for my follow-up exam. We started off with a CT scan, then headed to the doctor's office. I felt good. I felt confident. I knew he was going to tell me that my fracture was all healed, and I could be done with the brace.

The doctor came into the room with a computer on a rolling table, saying, "Yeah, pretty standard. These things normally take about three months to heal."

I was stunned. I wasn't healed? It confused me.

"I? Still?" The words weren't making it out. "I still need to wear the brace."

"Yes, your neck is still broken. But the great news is that everything stayed well aligned, so you don't have to have surgery to realign things."

I was shocked and stunned with disbelief. Surely, this couldn't be right.

"Have you ever seen a CT scan? Come look at this."

He logged in to his computer and pulled up images of my neck. To my amazement, he was able to create a visual 3-D rendering of my neck. He showed us the front, back, and sides. Then, he flipped the view, and we could see through the vertebra.

It was broken, fully broken. Your cervical vertebrae are kind of shaped like a fidget spinner. One whole prong was completely broken off of the body of the vertebra. Miraculously, it had stayed perfectly aligned, causing no damage to the nearby nerves and muscles.

Looking at this imaging of my spine, I realize for the first time that my facet joint was broken. Previously, I thought that a *fracture* was some sort of crack, some sort of lesser break. This image before me showed that I wasn't messing with any small crack in a bone. One third of my vertebra was sitting on the other side of a thick black line, a break in the bone.

The image below is one of many from my CT scan that day. Notice how the vertebra looks like a "V" wearing a hat. Over on the right, toward the top of the "V" there is a black line. That is my break.

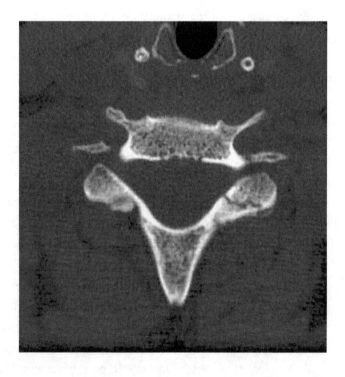

"See this black line. When that line is gray and fuzzy, it's healing. Do you see how yours is all black?"

My mouth was dry. "Yes."

"Yeah, it still has a lot of healing to do. Hopefully, you'll be all set at the end of your three months."

Hopefully? I hadn't believed that I would have to wear this neck brace for the full three months, and now I was learning that I might have to wear it for even longer. My head was spinning.

"Alright. Let's take a look and make sure that your brace is set up so that your facet joint will heal correctly." The doctor gestured for me to take a seat again.

He came up, looked me over, pulled on the knob in the center of my neck brace and gave it a spin, lifting my chin higher. The sudden, dramatic movement made my neck muscles seize up and spasm. "There. That looks better. People always have a tough time getting their neck braces correctly aligned."

"You were the one who set it when I was in the hospital. I haven't adjusted it since." I was ready to leave and starting to lose my cool. Thankfully, he left and the nurse came in to schedule another visit for us at the end of September. I was able to calm down and make some jokes with her.

My husband and I left the hospital and quickly walked to his truck. I buckled myself in, and then I fell apart and immediately started sobbing. Disappointment leaves a particularly bitter taste in your mouth, especially when you don't see it coming.

I did my best to get myself under control for the drive home. When we were back home, I politely went upstairs, grabbed my own box of tissues, and had a full-on, adult-sized fit in the privacy of my own bedroom.

I don't get upset about things very often, and I never throw tantrums. However, I have a solid rule to protect my emotional wellbeing. I am allowed to feel any feeling for at least five minutes.

If I think that it's ridiculous for me to feel that way, I still go ahead. More often than not, I get tired of the emotions that don't serve me and stop my pity party before my five minutes are up.

Today was different, though. Today, I had so many feelings to process—sadness, depression, self-pity, and anger. How could I have left myself so vulnerable? Why didn't I consider that I might have to keep wearing my neck brace? I certainly didn't do myself a service by putting on my blinders and living in a haze of optimism.

Still, when my five minutes were up, I threw away my soggy tissues, wiped my tears, and moved forward with my day.

Dealing with Stress

15

August 10, 2017

I t's my older son's back-to-school night. With the chance of rain in the forecast, and my desire to not be a pedestrian during the back-to-school craziness, I arranged for my sister-in-law and her family to pick us up. I'm so grateful that my older son will be going to elementary school with two of his cousins. They arrive, and we load into the car with our supplies and head to the school a block away from our house.

Truthfully, back-to-school night is the closest I have come to "losing it" in public. The chaos of the St. Louis City Museum has nothing on my son's elementary school gathering. I'm so worried about someone bumping into me or me bumping into someone. Plus, with the fast movement and my inability to move my head, I know my reaction time is quite poor. I would not be able to stop myself from falling this time.

Carefully, I steer my kids to my older son's kindergarten room. Thankfully, I'm friends with one of his teachers, so she already knows about my broken neck. Truthfully, with the stress of sending my baby off to kindergarten, I don't know if I could have told the story to a stranger without breaking down and crying.

In times like these, I like to think about one of my favorite movies, *What About Bob?* I turn to Dr. Leo Marvin's wise words and *baby step* myself through the situation. *Baby step* unload the backpack. *Baby step* talk to the teacher. *Baby step* find your son's name at the table. *Baby step* fill out the information they need. Now, get the hell out of there! That last part isn't from Dr. Marvin—it's from me.

Quickly, we make our way outside. With my indoor duties done, I feel so much better being outside…at last. I had dropped off all of my older son's supplies for kindergarten, and I hadn't fallen apart. It was like a burden had been lifted from my shoulders.

With my stresses gone, I feel more able to be myself. I sign my son up for school lunches although we plan on bringing his lunch, and I sign up for PTA. Gotta love those people who rush by the PTA table, saying, "Oh, I don't think I have the time" or "Oh, I work."

I'm sure I was silently laughing. Once or twice, I almost turned around and replied, "Oh, honey! They don't want you. They want your $6. Do you have $6?" I didn't because that would be rude. Plus, that's probably not the first impression I want to give to other parents.

But, it's the truth. If anyone asks you to join PTA, they need your check. They'll call if they need anything else, and you can tell them "No" then. But, for now, they need a small amount of money.

Signing up for the PTA entitled us to free hot dogs and lemonade. For my sons and me, that's about the best summertime meal ever. The only way they could sweeten the pot would be to have chocolate milk shakes later. We make our way to the hot dogs and lemonade, taking one of each, and then we move over to the side to eat.

While we are eating, I see one of my friends. Through Facebook, she knows that I broke my neck, but she hasn't seen me since then. It is nice talking to her and her daughter. For some reason, with the stress of going into the school now behind me, I feel much more at ease.

However, I did also feel like a freak. The kids were fine and hardly looked me. They were so happy to see their friends and find out who was in which classes. It was different with the parents, though. I felt the weight of their stares. I imagined they were thinking things like: *What the hell happened to her?*

Without the confinement of the school walls, it feels easier to shrug off the stares. Still, the whole process constantly reiterates how badly I want this collar off…and now I know it will be seven more weeks.

After our hot dogs are gone, my sister-in-law drives us home. Inside, the boys and I cuddle on the couch. Sometimes, the little one and I watch something on his tablet. Sometimes, the older one and I play Minecraft. It was a great ending to a day that could have been very stressful.

August 11, 2017

Three clients in a row didn't used to feel like a lot of work. Sure, when I was pregnant, I took more breaks. I would see two people, then break to go to the bathroom and eat a snack. Now, though, I'm mentally exhausted. I don't feel like writing.

Mostly, I feel like vegging out in front of the TV, exercising, or sleeping. I suppose I could just sit and watch TV or decide to take a nap at a random time of the day, but I do want to be productive. Plus, I don't want to get out of the habit of working.

That just leaves exercise, and although I can go for a walk or use my treadmill, other forms of exercising are pretty much off the table. I sure wish they weren't because my body feels crummy. I miss yoga. I know I've gained weight, and I want to exercise to get off the extra pounds. Mind you, I don't want to quit eating my ice cream or drinking my chocolate milk. I have to have some pick-me-ups, for heaven's sake.

My frustration rolls through me like depression. This is stupid. I go over to the studio and get out The Orb massage ball. I love The Orb! It's a foam massage ball with a little bit of grip to the surface. This helps breakup adhesions right below the skin's surface.

I start rolling along my tight spots. I roll my lower body—my hamstrings, calves, glutes, piriformis, adductors, and quadriceps. I work especially hard on the dent on the front of my left thigh. When I'm done rolling, I'm not sure that the dent in my quad is gone, but my whole body feels a lot better.

Next, I get the tennis balls and go for my low back and psoas. I lie down on my back and try to get comfortable. Then, I place a tennis ball on each side of my spine at my bottom ribs. This is where the psoas starts. I hold and breathe. As I breathe, I feel tension leave. *Things will be better,* I think. *I feel better.*

I roll from my bottom rib down to my glutes, stopping every inch or so to let the tennis balls do their work on my tight body. I think I'm going to start doing this every day.

If I can commit to rolling out my tight muscles, I will at least feel better. If I feel better, I should be in a better mood and have more energy. Plus, if my muscles aren't so tight, maybe I can figure out a way to safely incorporate more movement and exercise into my day. It will be a trick, but I think I can do it.

The Food Funnel 16

August 12, 2017

This is so odd, and I don't know why I haven't mentioned it until now, but when I eat, I tuck a paper towel into the edge of my neck brace. We lovingly refer to it as my "food funnel." Early on, I discovered that lots of food fell into my neck brace.

Imagine, if you will, a woman eating M&Ms. She misses her mouth, as she frequently did even when she wasn't wearing a neck brace. What becomes of the M&M? Does it bounce off and fall onto the floor somewhere?

No. It slides like a freaking Plinko chip from *The Price Is Right*, slipping to the left just as I'm about to grab it and dropping to the right as I touch it, each time escaping the grasp of my frantic fingers. Clumsily, I fumble for the M&M until it is too late. My fingertips can no longer feel it, and I wonder, *Where is it?*

After a shift and wiggle, it *shoots out of my neck hole.* That's right, an M&M shoots from the center of my neck brace. It doesn't help that the hole in the middle of the neck brace makes it look like I maybe have also received a tracheotomy of some sorts. So, I'm wearing this brace that looks like I've also had a tracheotomy, and an M&M shoots out—like I have just shot something out of my new blowhole.

After the initial M&M incident, I decided to use a paper towel to help catch my food. Literally, I have lifted the far end of the paper towel to help guide rejected food into my mouth. Hence the name "food funnel."

Using a paper towel or napkin this way helps keep my neck brace clean. The protective covering keeps the white part of the neck brace white, and I also have a quick place to wipe my fingers. My kids also find this very convenient. In the past, they have wiped their hands and even their noses on me. Now, with my handy paper towel, they use that instead.

Because of this, I have started wearing the paper towel for slightly extended periods of time. For example, if the youngest is eating, I will wear my paper towel. The kid is a grazer, so I can sometimes wear my paper towel for hours.

This has developed into an issue of sorts for me. I have found that I will regularly have slight panic attacks before meeting with my clients because I can't tell if I'm still wearing my paper towel. It's not difficult to find out; I simply reach up with my hand and feel. I am slightly worried, however, that since I have become accustomed to the neck brace, I could also become accustomed to wearing the paper towel—and that would certainly be weird.

Yesterday, I committed to rolling my body on The Orb so I would feel better. Today, I followed through by rolling again. I feel so much better. Plus, the whole time I was rolling, I was talking on the phone with one of my best friends. *Hooray* for feeling better physically and emotionally.

Facing the Consequences of Bad Decisions

17

August 13, 2017

L ast night, I worked on my computer while sitting in bed. Unlike other times, I didn't prop my computer up on my lap or on pillows. I worked for only about half an hour, and the topic wasn't too stressful, so it didn't seem likely that my shoulders would get tense. However, by the time I shut my laptop, my neck and head *hurt so bad*. For the first time in a long while, I had to take acetaminophen.

I took my pills, went to bed, and shifted. Everything hurt. My collar felt like it was choking me. Once, I yawned so big that my chin slipped beneath the edge of the collar and was caught. There was a moment of panic, a twinge of pain, and I figured out that I could close my mouth—crisis averted. By the time it was bedtime, everything felt difficult and like a chore.

In the middle of the night, the younger one kept hopping into our bed, and my husband kept snoring. Finally, I made my way to our guest bed. With no distractions, my mind was able to settle, and I finally went back to sleep.

Tonight, when I go to bed, I will not write with my computer on my bed. Maybe I'll prop it up or stand while I write. Maybe I won't write at all. Regardless, I'm not going to put myself in the same situation again that might cause me pain.

In the morning, we had breakfast plans with our brother-in-law and his family—including his parents and best friend. It's not as oblique as it sounds. We're a tight group, and the same people who were there for breakfast are always invited to our kids' birthday parties.

Everyone decided to go outside to play. After some very fun time on a big rope/tire swing, and at least two verbal warnings that the swing is much heavier than it looks, the kids hopped off. As my older son tried to stop the swing, it blasted him in the face, hitting him on the bridge of his nose. I was sure he would have two black eyes. The poor guy.

I saw the tire swing coming at him and had yelled for him to get back as it popped him in the face, knocking his head back, and sending him to the ground. To his credit, he says that he decided to sit on the ground so that it wouldn't hit him in the face anymore. I told him that was a good idea. The rope burn/scuff mark goes from his left tear duct to the bottom tip of his right nostril. We put ice on it right away.

As soon as it hit him, I was on my way to him. I know I'm not supposed to run, but I ran to him. I grabbed his hand (because I'm not allowed to lift him with my broken neck) and led him to a chair. My poor, sweet boy. He climbed onto my lap, and I held him, and we rocked.

Later, I told my husband that he needed to keep a close eye on the two-year-old. If we go into the ER with me in a neck brace, our older son with a newly beaten face, and our younger son with any sorts of injuries, they're going to take my husband away—*and he's our ride!*

After my older son's accident, everyone decided to play baseball. As a family, we don't quite have enough people to make two teams, but we do pretty well. It was such a joy to watch my older son get a good hit and run the bases. Ultimately, he was tagged out at home, but I was proud.

Somehow, his minor success made my broken neck seem not so bad...like it was okay that I broke my neck because I instilled some baseball knowledge and skill. However, I know that's not the truth because I know that everything he knows about baseball, he learned by watching the movie, *The Sandlot*. Since the two-year-old has insisted on watching *The Sandlot* one to three times a day, we have all learned about baseball. Honestly, I think it has taught them a love for baseball, not to judge people because of their athletic abilities, and the importance of a good group of friends. At least, that's what I hope it's teaching them.

Later that night, my older son wanted to practice riding his bike without the training wheels. He's been working on it, and it's been tough, but he's been a trouper.

One time after he crashed I said, "Do you remember when we were trying to find a bike for Mom?"

"Yeah."

"Do you remember when I crashed into that trash can in front of all those shops? Or when I crashed into the glass of that one business?"

"Yeah."

"That was pretty funny, wasn't it?"

"Yeah," he laughed.

"And each time, I got up and kept going. You're doing a great job. I'm proud of you."

He took off riding, and that night, he mastered the rounding of the corners, which is something I still have on my to-do list. He did seven full loops on our driveway without having to stop once. I am fully impressed.

August 14, 2017

I started a walking and stretching regime. I hope I'm making a good decision about adding stretching before and after walking. I think I am.

August 15, 2017

On a walk today, a butterfly actually flew into my neck hole and give me butterfly kisses on my throat. It's not as magical and lovely as you may imagine. In fact, it scared the heck out of me, and for some reason, I became afraid that it was going to fly into my mouth.

The Beginning of Kindergarten and Changes for All of Us

18

August 16, 2017

Today was my older son's first day of kindergarten. He and I each cried only a little bit. Then, I came home and had one of the most productive days I've had in a long time. I tidied. I cleaned. I created a donation pile of clothes that I haven't worn in a while.

The whole time I did this, I was fully aware that it was because I didn't want to write. Right now, I'm working through the emotions that come with sending your baby to kindergarten. I think I'm handling it pretty well, but I don't want to add the stress of writing something helpful or meaningful while I try to work through my issues.

Although I'm glad that my son is growing up, it sure is hard to admit that he's as big as he is. In fact, this past week has been full of milestones. First, he learned to ride his bike without training wheels. Then, he didn't cry when he was hit in the face with a tire swing. This morning, when he woke up early, I asked him if he wanted to come get some snuggles, and he said, "No, I just want to get ready."

My baby is gone. In his place is a tall, skilled, Minecraft-loving guy. He's not my baby anymore. *He's a guy.*

I'll admit I felt good when he started to cry when we were leaving. At least he still needs us for something, although it doesn't always seem like it.

Once my husband left for work, I did what I suspect many stay at home moms do—I cleaned my house. Then, I basked in the cleanness all day long. No one spilled sticky things on the floor or tracked mud through the house.

Cleaning took about two hours. Then, I did something that I also think is very common—I started looking for a job. Mind you, I teach Pilates and yoga, plus I write for my website. However, I have actually been thinking about getting a job as an editor. I love reading other peoples' work and giving them constructive feedback. So, I did some online research and started working on a resume. I worry that because I've been out of the writing career field for so long, it will be difficult to get a job, but I hope not.

Honestly, with my broken neck and my older son starting kindergarten, I'm starting to feel a little emotional and kind of nuts. I swear, if I can't get a job editing, I may go crazy and decorate the house for Christmas once I can figure out how to get the tree upstairs. It's amazing how life changes can motivate you.

I had been thinking about looking for a freelance-editing job for months, but now I'm ready to take action. As I helped my husband edit his papers for his English 108 class, I felt pure joy.

While I read each paper, I questioned syntax, grammar, spelling, and punctuation. I taught my husband how to edit. Each time we talked about a topic, it sharpened my tools and directly improved my own writing. At least, I think it did. In any case, it felt like it did.

I looked for jobs online. I actually called about one local job. Then, I did something so crazy that I couldn't wait to tell my husband. I finally hooked up my computer at the desk that had been ready and waiting for me for over half a year. Crazy, right?

At our house, I have had my computer hooked up to an outlet on the side of our buffet. Then, I bring my computer over to the dining room table, and that's where I work. Today, though, I cleaned the desk, removing all the extraneous materials that had gathered on that horizontal surface. Then, I ran my power cord through my desk and carefully gathered all the cables together in one small area. I plugged in my computer, and it charged.

Maybe tomorrow I will actually sit at my desk and write.

August 17, 2017

Six weeks in, and six weeks until I'm done with this neck brace. I applied for my first editing job. I'm so excited! I hope I get it.

August 18, 2017

I'm trying to write a book, write for my website, get a job as a proofreader/copy editor, lose weight and build bone, all at the same time while dealing with all the emotions aroused by sending my first born to kindergarten. I'm exhausted.

Thankfully, my husband is working to lower his cholesterol, so I get to be healthier by default. That's the benefit of being lazy in the kitchen. If he wants to cook and eat healthy, I will probably not challenge him. Since I like having food passed to me (instead of preparing it myself), I should be able to be healthier in these next few months.

This morning, my son and I walked the block to school. Then, I came back and had a client. Right after my client, an old friend came for a walk, bringing her baby along. We walked my old practice route from when I used to run 5ks, so we walked over three miles.

When I came back from the walk, my husband had made these healthy smoothies. It was very green and smelled fresh. My philosophy is that if I can take shots, I can drink anything. Luckily, I didn't need to talk myself through drinking this. It tasted pretty good, and I felt like a champ knowing that I was ingesting the benefits from multiple fruits and vegetables.

I know I should eat better, particularly during this challenging time when I'm healing. However, ice cream, chocolate milk, and quesadillas are so freaking delicious. Wednesday night, I made chicken nuggets, mac and cheese, and green beans for dinner. That night, the kids and I all had tons of sinus drainage and boogers. No question about it: there's a correlation between personal health and what you're eating.

Ugh, now that I've just written that, I suppose it won't be too long before I'll be back to eating Paleo, which means no more ice cream, chocolate milk, quesadillas, or mac and cheese for me.

August 19, 2017

What a productive day. I worked with a client, posted two articles, and successfully completed a quiz for an employment website.

As I was telling my client, 12 weeks in the cervical collar means 84 days. If I write a page of content every day, and then include my physical therapy time, I should technically have enough pages for a legitimate book.

Man, that would be so great to write this book, print it, and have people read it. If it helped *only one person with a broken neck*, I would feel successful.

How strange success is. Why do we have the need to feel successful? And what does success even mean? It's not a constant. One person's success is probably another person's failure.

More importantly, I suppose I need to seriously start on my self-work to figure out what I'm needing. I feel like something is missing. Being a mom is important and so is helping people get rid of pain, but I can tell that I'm still searching for something else. I'll do my best to leave myself open to new possibilities and see what I discover.

Right now, I'm missing the day dates that my husband and I used to go on when the kids were at the sitter on Mondays. Between him working on his days off and me trying to catch up on my website content for the month, we haven't been able to go out since we were on vacation. I do need some alone time with my man.

That won't be in our future this week, though. Monday is the solar eclipse, so we'll have both boys at home with us to watch it. Plus, a couple friends will be in from Kansas City. I look forward to this memorable moment and am so thankful that we live in one of the top viewing spots in the country. However, I wouldn't mind a little quality time with my husband and some good food.

August 20, 2017

I had terrible dreams last night. In fact, I've been having terrible dreams all week. Honestly, I thought that once I applied for work to be an editor or proofreader, my bad dreams would stop. In fact, since I have been applying for jobs, they have become worse.

Plus, my self-esteem is quite low right now. Every ignored application feels like a slap to the face and a snicker behind my back. *Like I'd hire her! Why would she think she's qualified for this?* Those are the questions I imagine they ask as they read my application showing a 15-year gap from writing.

Personally, I wonder if I'm crumbling under this pressure because I haven't practiced yoga in such a long time. I know that well-crafted practices can improve your thoughts and feelings. However, in my attempt to completely heal and follow the doctor's orders, I haven't practiced yoga since my accident—almost two months.

Today, I'm going to try to straddle the line between following my doctor's orders and practicing yoga. I'm going to try to complete a nice standing/hip opening practice. I've already picked a sequence out from one of my favorite yogis, Bruce Bowditch. Somehow, he has such a way of stringing together poses to get the absolute most benefit that they have to offer.

I'm in my tank top and shorts and, after I write, I'm going to practice. Actually, after I write and drink my special cholesterol-reducing breakfast drink, I will practice.

My husband has taken to making us breakfast smoothies. I have no idea what goes into this thing, but it completely tastes like the color green and the adjective "healthy." Aside from that, I have no idea how to describe the taste. There's flax seed, so there's a sort of a gritty crunch to it. Once, I saw a mango go in, but I didn't think we had mangoes in the house, so I don't know if that's in today's drink.

I know that spinach isn't in it because I cooked up the rest of it for dinner last night. Spinach is one of my favorite vegetables to prepare because you can cook the crap out of it, and it tastes exactly the same as if you cooked it perfectly. As long as you don't let the oil and garlic burn, you're good to go.

Today's drink is definitely not as good as yesterday's because of the lack of spinach. At least it's not as bad as when he snuck a banana into our oatmeal. That was terrible, and I was tempted to tell him so, but since I don't like making food for myself, I decided I wouldn't rock the boat.

Oh my gosh! This just occurred to me. He bought a kale blend the other day. Maybe there's kale in here. Ugh, that would explain why it's not as good. Man, I hope he's not sneaking me kale.

*****

We went to my favorite ice cream shop today. Normally, we do the drive-thru, but we needed to grab beers and ice for a family party and, since our ice cream shop is attached to a convenience store, we went in. We ordered, and I patiently waited for our shakes while my husband purchased the other supplies.

While I hung out at the counter, another couple came in behind me. They were looking over the menu and seemed to be getting ready to order, so I scooted over. All of a sudden, in walked a guy who was also rockin' the Aspen Vista neck brace.

"Twins!" I yelled, pointing at our matching cervical collars.

"Yeah. Surgery?" asked the older gentleman.

"No. I broke it." I replied. "You?"

"Surgery. They took out my C4. Which vertebra for you?"

"C6."

At this point, the other couple completely ceded their space in line, allowing the gentleman and I to stand by each other and talk. It turns out he had neck surgery a couple of days after I broke my neck, we both have about six weeks left of the neck brace, and we have the same doctor.

This was my first sighting of someone else in a neck brace since breaking my own neck. It was thrilling to find someone in my same boat. His wife had to drive him to get ice cream, just like my husband had to drive me. He had to suffer through the summer heat just like I did. I'm sure when he went out or went to parties, he got the same stares, the same questions. We might have technically been strangers, but we were tied to each other on a much deeper level. Others might have sympathy for our situation, but we had empathy for each other, and that boosts your relationship to a whole new level.

My shakes were ready, so we wished each other happy healing. As I started to head out, I noticed that the other couple let him go ahead and order. That was nice of them.

August 21, 2017

Eclipse Day! I obviously don't know where you were on Eclipse Day, but I was in the #2 city in the U.S. to view the eclipse. That's right, good old St. Joseph, Missouri was named the second best place to watch the eclipse. I think some place in Oregon earned the #1 spot.

I have no idea what made us a better place to view the eclipse. In fact, it took me some time to realize the absurdity of the whole ranking situation. For example, because people were making such a big deal about us being ranked #2, I thought we would have great reasons, a particular edge, over why people should watch the eclipse in St. Joseph and not, say, Kansas City.

Kansas City is about an hour south of us. For whatever reason, I thought they would have an inferior experience until I saw the bandwidth for eclipse viewing. It was a stripe almost as wide as the Midwest itself that swept all the way across the country.

You know what the viewing difference was in St. Joseph versus Kansas City? St. Joseph was projected as having a 2 minute 38 second stretch of totality. Kansas City would have only 1 minute 48 seconds.

What is happening in your life that you so badly need the extra 50 seconds of darkness? Yet, people were planning to come to St. Joseph. Rational people and friends of mine were planning to come up for the day.

I'm sure the idea was to have an event to celebrate this monumental moment in natural history and celebrate with family and friends for, well, 50 seconds longer than you would have at home. My friends, though, bailed as soon as they saw reports indicating that anyone wanting to come to St. Joseph from Kansas City should plan on leaving the house by 4 a.m. in order to be in town in time for the full-eclipse process.

I don't blame them. I can't mentally justify spending hours in thick traffic in order to see an extra 50 seconds of pitch black. Maybe I'm missing the point. It's possible. I didn't read any of the hype or explanation for why we were selected and elevated to such a high rank on a list of cities.

In truth, it was an honor just to be nominated.

Although I had been regularly checking the weather reports, I still wasn't prepared for our Eclipse Day weather—rain. Rain, like no other.

It was overcast when we woke up. *Good*, I thought. *Let's get this rain over with*. Unfortunately, it didn't work that way. It rained. Then, it was overcast. We started to go on a walk during the eclipsing process, but it started raining—again.

It rained during the whole eclipsing process. If you weren't anal-retentively looking out your window like we were, you might have thought that it rained through the entire eclipse. Luckily, it didn't. As the sky darkened, the rain stopped. It was so black outside during totality, like 11 p.m. on a night with no moon, when it was actually 1:10 in the afternoon.

We went outside and watched some of our neighbors shoot off fireworks. No one needed any special glasses because the cloud cover was so extreme.

Then, just like that, the moon scooched over, and a sliver of bright silvery sun shined over everything. Immediately, we were moving back to daytime. As the clouds moved, we could occasionally glimpse the partially covered sun. It was fantastic.

We decided to finish our walk. Right as we returned home, it started raining again.

I'm not joking. I cannot remember a day in the past few years when it has rained so much. The eclipse was amazing, but what gets me is that if everyone in St. Joseph were asked to name a date when it rained, I think everyone would say Eclipse Day.

It's so rare to get everyone in a community to pay attention to the weather outside. We all have different lives, different jobs, and different perspectives. However, in my community at least, we were unified with this thought: *How dare it rain on Eclipse Day?*

Big News from Preschool and the Hardest Test I've Ever Taken

19

August 22, 2017

Today was productive. The family rode together to take the younger son to school. Then, my husband and I walked our older son to his school. I love being able to walk him to school. The school is quite close to our house. From our front porch, we can see the playground and parking lot.

This makes diving my son to school on a warm morning feel quite ridiculous. Sitting in traffic is annoying and, as we look for a parking place so that we can walk him in, I inevitably feel like a jerk when I get out of the car, turn, and see our house in the near distance. Plus, our short walk means that we also get to visit with and hug my sixth-grade niece (our crossing guard) before her school day begins.

I was so proud of my big kindergartner. He cried only a little bit today, and he didn't try to have a death grip on me as we entered the building. He's come a long way in a short amount of time.

After drop-off, *three hours of freedom* until we pick the little one up from preschool. I especially enjoy these days when my husband is at home. It's so great to be able to talk to him and hang out.

Normally, we don't do much, but I feel like we're getting to talk to each other and be there for each other when he's at home in the mornings.

Throughout the day, I applied for several proofreader jobs and wrote four articles for my website. I needed a productive day because they help boost my self-esteem and happiness level. There's nothing quite as satisfying as getting a task checked off your to-do list.

Then, we got a great surprise when we picked our younger son up from preschool. The teacher walked him out to the car and told us that he had pottied at preschool. As a parent of a two-year-old, this is just about the very best news you will have all day, maybe all week. As a parent with a broken neck, the potential for ditching diapers (and the pain and awkwardness that come with changing them) brings an almost overwhelming joy.

"Does he do this at home?" his teacher asked.

"Yes, he's been using the potty some at home."

"Whatever rewards you use, send some along. We're happy to use your reward system."

"I let him dump his pee into the toilet. That's all. That's all he needs."

"Well, we don't have that here. They use a seat to sit on a low toilet."

"He's good then."

God bless this low-maintenance boy. Ditching diaper-duty was just the gift I wanted while healing my broken neck.

We went home, took a nap, and then walked to get my older son from school. I worked while my husband started getting dinner ready and, by the time he was done, my whole workday was complete. We ate dinner, took a walk, and the boys rode their bikes.

August 23, 2017

Much like my other days this week, I have been productive. I helped drop off both boys and witnessed tearless departures in both cases. Then, I came home and took an AP editing quiz on my online job site.

I knew the quiz would be tough. A thousand people had passed it, while over four thousand had taken the test. That's lofty. Despite the fact that I have not edited anything with AP style in mind since the very early 2000s, I was confident that I would do well on the test. I grabbed my AP stylebook (from 1999), a couple pieces of peanut butter toast, some chocolate milk, and settled in. *I've got this,* I thought.

At this point, I should know better than to think this thought. Every time I think, *Oh, I've got this,* things epically fail. For example, there was this one time I thought I'd teach my boys how to play baseball in the backyard. You know what happened next.

My hesitation, pause, and utter uncertainty at the first question made me literally start sweating. Seriously! If you were editing in AP style, you'd look your questions up in your book. Why does this quiz exist? But, if I could figure out a way to pass, that would look good in my online work profile.

With my trusty, possibly outdated book, I plugged through the questions. Naturally, I tried my hardest to answer correctly and do my best. Sometimes, I knew the answer immediately, though, and this gave me a boost of confidence.

After thirty-odd minutes, I finished the test. It seemed like the scoring process took forever. Scoring. Scoring. Scoring. *Is my Wi-Fi actually working?* Scoring. And finally, a quiz about how complete and correct I thought the quiz was. *What? It's fine. How'd I do?*

The next screen answered my question: I passed! I earned a 3.4 out of 5 and ranked 388 out of, well, however many people had passed. Not only that, I received a special banner that said I was in the top 10 percent on that test.

For a moment, my jaw opened, which is quite a feat since the neck brace pretty much keeps my mouth closed at all times. Inside my head, I imagined that my jaw dropped, and I looked like the painting, "The Scream." In fact, I think the voice in my head did scream.

Truly, I was amazed. I felt like reporters should start hounding my door. *How does it feel, passing the most ridiculous quiz ever? And finishing in the top 10 percent. You must be some sort of editing genius.*

That didn't happen of course, but my husband congratulated me and, after he left for work, I took myself out for a fantastically long walk. I called my best friend. There is truly no one in the world like your best friend. Talking with her on the phone made an hour-long walk fly by in an instant. I walked over three miles, and I would have kept going if she hadn't had to get off the phone.

I returned home and was about to go film some videos for my website when I decided that I should take my hot and sweaty self to the tub. I know people wouldn't be able to smell me through the screen, but I felt like I looked sweaty. I started the water and added some bubbles.

Is there anything more luxurious than taking a bubble bath in the middle of the day with no one else in the house? I think not. It was magnificent—everything I always remembered it to be. I soaked. I exfoliated. I shaved my legs.

This is a very big deal for a gal with a broken neck. Leg shaving is quite tricky when you have to bend at the waist to see what's going on. Naturally, sitting in a hot tub and manhandling your leg to help it rotate the direction you need is the better, safer way for hair removal instead of trying to bend forward in the shower. It's much safer to sit and lift your leg toward you.

After my bath, I filmed three videos. I also wrote the articles to accompany two of the videos and picked up both boys. When I came home, my husband was cooking dinner, which was fantastic.

I accomplished so much, and I didn't have to make any dinner. Those are my favorite days.

Embrace Healing

20

August 28, 2017

I didn't want to break my neck, but I did. It was an accident. The sequence of events could have gone any number of ways and created a multitude of results, but it didn't. It only happened one way.

When I think through all the possible results, my present situation is one of the best. To have my neck break and stay perfectly aligned with no pain, weakness, or numbness is a miracle. In this one accident, I think I've used up "all nine lives" and called in all my favors simultaneously. Despite my seemingly good fortune, I'm not always happy.

Having a broken neck hasn't been fun. Sometimes, it's frustrating and annoying. But you know what? I could be dead, so I try not to complain. Instead, I turn to my yoga practice.

Intention

In yoga, whenever I'm in a difficult pose, I return to my intention that I set at the beginning of practice. I often try to keep my intentions very simple so I won't forget them later. Some of my intentions have been: *have fun* or *lift out of your hips*.

These days, the intention that I set when I get out of bed is: Embrace healing.

With my restricted activities, I'm not practicing yoga poses, but that doesn't mean I have to quit practicing yoga. Yoga is so much more than just poses that simultaneously challenge your body and help it feel better.

For me, yoga extends to my attitude and my philosophy regarding my personal code of conduct. Yoga helps me embrace the changes in my life and to grit my teeth and lean into the challenges.

Lean Into It

I still vividly remember days in the past when I've had a challenging yoga practice. It seemed like every posture was designed to annoy or taunt me. Then, they were all strung together one after another, seemingly trying to break me.

Instead of becoming frustrated or annoyed, I would lean into the experience. I would turn to my intention and say it over and over: *Have fun. Have fun. Have fun.* I would repeat my intention until I was finally taking my own advice.

Truthfully, it reminds me of the part in the movie, *What About Bob?* when Bob tells himself, "I feel good; I feel great; I feel wonderful." Over and over again, he says the exact same thing. Sometimes, he changes the inflection of his voice to assert to himself that he does mean what he is saying.

That's what an intention is. It's a few words that give you strength and have a personal meaning—words that can help you rise up out of a bad place and move past the discomfort of your present situation.

When you find yourself recovering from something, whether physical or emotional trauma, I invite you to embrace healing. Lean into the discomfort and know that you will emerge a stronger person.

The Mice

21

August 29, 2017

Today was a wonderful day. My husband was off work, I was productive, and I snuggled with my little one. It should have been a good night. I should have slept well, but I didn't.

While I was sleeping, I heard this little scratching noise. At first, I thought it might be one of the cats digging at something. Then, I realized the noise was right behind my head. It scared the bejeezus out of me, and I sprung from bed. I turned on my lamp, ready to catch the mouse-culprit, only to find nothing.

That's not true. I found a disgruntled husband who thought I was crazy.

"They're in the wall. Turn off your lamp and go to bed, Sarah."

I turned off the lamp and climbed in bed, but I couldn't go to sleep. The noises seemed so loud. It was like something was squeaking and scratching right behind my ear.

I hopped up and started knocking where I heard them digging. The mice didn't care. They didn't stop, and they didn't switch locations. They kept on doing whatever they were doing while I waited for them to stop so I could go back to sleep.

It was a long wait. I hate mice.

Two Months Since My Fall

22

August 30, 2017

Whenever I see friends and family, they ask, "How's your neck healing?" It's so kind of them to ask, but without a CT scan, I have no real way of knowing for sure how I'm healing. I feel like a goofball answering, "Good, I guess," but it's the only completely accurate answer I can give. Here's where I am in the healing process right now.

My Neck

My neck is still broken, but I've finally mentally adjusted to the fact that my facet joint was completely broken. I took time to mentally adjust, and now I'm counting down the days. In about a month, I should get the all-clear to be done with my neck brace.

My Face

About six weeks after I lost half my eyebrow, it's all back. I'm very pleased with how well the eyebrow hair has grown back, but I wonder how long it will take the scar tissue to bust up. Previously, I believed the scar tissue caused an odd sensitivity to cool breezes from the car air conditioner and our ceiling fan, but I haven't had any issues with scar sensitivity recently. Hopefully, that odd pain is gone for good.

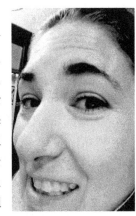

My Right Knee

You might remember that my right knee was skinned so badly that they did an X-ray to make sure that my patellar tendon was still attached. It was, and the wound healed faster than I thought it would.

Now, I'm doing my best to lighten the scar tissue. Every so often, I exfoliate to remove dead skin. Every day, I use a coconut oil-based body oil, and I have seen a noticeable reduction in the size and darkness of my scar.

Despite my jokes and nonchalant attitude, this was a very serious injury. In fact, it wasn't until this week, nearly nine weeks since the accident, that I was able to kneel with both knees on a padded surface. I still can't kneel on our floors, which are mostly hardwood and tile. However, I can kneel on my boys' beds to kiss them goodnight—a huge win in my book.

My Left Thigh

My left thigh seemed to be the simplest of my injuries, but it has proven to be the most challenging. When I fell, I banged my left thigh on the side of our wooden back step. Within a few days, I had a substantial bruise that continued to grow each day for weeks. The largest it ever became was slightly bigger than the palm of my hand.

Over time, the bruise went away and left a four-inch long, half-inch wide dent. I'm hoping the dent in my thigh has something to do with fascia. To try to remove my ding, I drink plenty of water to hydrate the injured muscle, and I roll on The Orb, trying to remove any myofascial adhesions that may be creating the dent.

Although I haven't noticed the dent decrease in size, I'm going to keep rolling the area to see if I can improve it. Even if rolling won't get rid of my dent, it improves the health and functionality of my leg muscles.

The Decision to Go Sugar-Free

23

September 3, 2017

I decided to quit eating sugar. Why the heck did I decide to quit eating sugar? Today has been difficult, and I really needed some chocolate right now. However, I kept it together, didn't eat any sugar for the whole day, had only moderate headaches and anger issues, and didn't eat the ice cream that I had been craving all day long

I can tell you this much—I had better lose some weight.

September 4, 2017

I woke up, determined to continue my sugar-free quest. By lunchtime, I had kissed those hopes goodbye. My husband made me a sandwich for lunch. It happens that the only kind of bread I like to eat has sugar. Go figure. What a surprise.

I ate the sandwich and prepared for the birthday party we were about to attend. My sister-in-law has removed many foods from her family's pantry in a quest to improve behavioral issues. She has had great success, to the extent that my nephew could greatly reduce his ADD medications. Naturally, I figured that the birthday party would have many sugar-free options.

However, I did not count on them providing cookie cake and regular sugar ice cream. I had some of each and noted that neither actually tasted as good as I thought it would. This made me a little upset. How dare they not be the most fantastic thing I've ever eaten in my life! I broke my sugar-free streak of, okay, two hours this time, but still, these foods should have been superb.

Fortunately, I was able to hop into my sister-in-law's hot tub with the boys. We didn't have the jets turned on, so the bottom pad of my collar just barely got wet. It was amazing to sit in a pool of sorts. In fact, it was the only time I've been in the water since I broke my neck.

When I was a kid, I was a pool bum. I was on the swim team and took additional lessons. As a teenager, I was one of the girls who read a book while she tanned. Whenever I was hot, I'd get in the water to cool off, then go back to reading.

I cherish these memories. When I reflect on this time in my life, I think about how relaxed I was by the pool. I think about how I'd get a nice, warm tan; then come home and take a nap on the couch. I'd get up, shower, eat, and go out for the night…it was magical. Every time that I get to swim at a pool, I believe it helps me channel some locked-away part of the younger me. It helps me reconnect with who I used to be, and I find that very energizing.

Needless to say, with this neck brace being hot as hell and as super-absorbent as a maxi-pad, I haven't made my way into the water. Today, though, was different. It seemed like the perfect time to hop into a hot tub.

Only my boys and I were allowed in. Everyone else had been in the pond or was covered in soap for the slip-n-slide. Not us, though. We held out for the hot tub, and it paid off.

Just the three of us were floating, laughing, and kind of swimming in our own private pool. It was wonderful. I reconnected with my younger self. Everything felt right with the world, like I'm right where I need to be, like this broken neck is perfect timing." Now, mind you, I have no idea why this break is perfect timing. However, I had a strong feeling everything was working according to plan and turning out in my favor.

God bless you, Universe, if that ends up being the truth.

September 5, 2017

I was so tired today. I'm not sure what is going on, but my productivity definitely decreased today. I'm going to sleep.

September 6, 2017

I woke up very motivated and had another great day. Yesterday's slump must have been a fluke. Maybe I overdid it somehow, and my body was exhausted.

By dinnertime, I had a different opinion. I think I'm getting a cold. After a wonderful day, I'm feeling crummy. I sure hope this isn't a cold.

Living with a Cold and a Neck Brace

24

September 8, 2017

Yes, I have a cold. I feel like junk. To soothe my spirit, I watched some of the movie *Top Gun* instead of working. Then, I rolled on The Orb and did a little Pilates/yoga routine. After I get over this cold, it's going to be time to build some core strength and muscle flexibility.

September 9, 2017

I am sick and very grateful that I didn't have a client scheduled for today. Still, I had a pretty good day with my kids while my husband worked. We decided we all wanted chicken nuggets. It was a bit of a struggle to find someone to pick up drive-thru lunch for us, but my older son has been doing so well at school, and that's what he wanted for lunch. I wanted to reward him. Plus, I watched two episodes of *Friends* and an episode of *The Price is Right*, so I feel pretty spoiled right now.

Sleeping with a Cold

Even without a broken neck, sleeping while you have a cold can be tricky at best and positively frustrating at its worst. Normally, I can get into bed on my back and adjust my head so I can breathe. It feels like positioning a TV antenna, but I can make small adjustments to the direction of my nose and, when I'm in the right spot, my sinus will open up, and I am able to breathe through one nostril.

Needless to say, that technique doesn't work with a broken neck. I decided to totally surrender to my cold, and I gathered the props needed for my very worst colds: a t-shirt and arthritis cream. When my colds are at their absolute worst and there's no way to adjust my nose to find an open sinus, I have a backup plan. I discovered that if I put a t-shirt over my nose and mouth, I could mouth-breathe and retain enough humidity so my nose, throat, and lips wouldn't dry out.

It's worth mentioning that, in the past, I experimented with several options before landing on a t-shirt. I tried cloth handkerchiefs and scarves, among other things. Long story short, the t-shirt provides enough weight to stay put, has enough size that you can move and still stay covered, is pliable enough to make a tent area, is sturdy enough to stay put after you make your tent, and is light enough that you don't feel like you're being smothered.

Now that you know what to do with your t-shirt, let me explain about the arthritis cream. When I was a kid, my folks would use a mentholated topical cream when I had a cold. This worked for a period of time; however, as I got older, it wasn't as effective. Maybe the cream was too old, or maybe my colds became too strong. Whatever the cause, it reached the point that if I held a jar of that stuff under my nose, my sinuses wouldn't clear.

Somehow, we stumbled upon arthritis cream, finding it would provide the same temporary heat and nostril-flaring smell. Because the arthritis cream packs more punch than the menthol cream, you have to be strategic in its placement. Here are the tricks that I've discovered through personal trial and error.

If your throat is sore, put some arthritis cream on your neck. Specifically, try to coat your lymph nodes on both sides of your neck, right under your jaw line. Those of us with a neck brace on need not do anything else. However, if your neck is not broken, I recommend you wrap a sock around your neck and secure it with a safety pin. I'm not joking. (Yeah, illness is pretty glamorous at my house.)

Another key area is on the chest. If you feel like you're getting a chest cold, smear some arthritis cream right on your breastbone. Wear a t-shirt to help keep the cream on your skin and prevent it from coming off on your sheets.

Finally, you can put arthritis cream on your face. I tend to put some on my temples, on the bridge of my nose, and right under each nostril—wherever you feel sinus pressure will work.

Be advised, I mentioned this one last because if you have to put cream on any of the other areas, you want to do them before this. Once you put this cream on your face, be ready to get to bed quickly and go to sleep. If you have other things to do, you will waste the effective period, won't get the maximal benefit to help you relax into sleep, and will notice that this hurts like hell. However, if you can fall asleep while it's helping to open your sinuses, you won't feel any pain at all.

Get in bed, put your t-shirt over your nose and mouth, and fall asleep.

September 10, 2017

I had a great morning with the kids. My husband took a short work call while the kids and I played. Then, he came back, and we all went for a walk. We had lunch together; the youngest and I napped together; I worked; and then, we went to family dinner with my in-laws. It was a very relaxing and pretty great day.

September 11, 2017

I decided to create an interview with myself about my broken neck. Essentially, this will end up being a fill-in-the-blank that I hope ends up reading more like an interview and less like a Mad Libs. You'll find my interview of myself on December 13, 2018 at the end of this book.

The Surprise 40th Birthday Party

September 15, 2017

Today is exciting. My husband and I are going to be part of a surprise 40th birthday destination celebration. His sister is turning 40 tomorrow, and her husband and another sister planned for a small group of us to celebrate in Hermann, Missouri.

If you're not familiar with Missouri, Hermann is a beautiful small town about an hour outside of St. Louis that is known for its wineries. Its beautiful downtown is located right on the river. The whole drive out, I can feel the excitement coursing through my veins.

First, though, we're going to drop our boys off at my parents' house. In order to make it to Hermann for dinner, we had to get our older one out of school a little early. Once we had him, all four of us were excited for our upcoming weekends. The boys were excited to spend time with Gram and Gramp, and my husband and I were excited to celebrate childfree for a weekend.

When we reached my parents' house, we hung out for a little bit and hopped back in the car for another hour ride. On our drive out to Hermann, a message from a stranger came through Facebook. A young woman had also broken her neck, and she wanted to thank me for my posts.

She said I was one of the only resources she could find about how to survive with a broken neck. Unlike me, this poor girl had a broken neck, broken leg, and broken spirits. I could tell she was suffering, and my heart went out to her. I chatted with her through Facebook messenger for part of our drive before we lost our connection.

Once we arrived in Hermann, we made our way to the bed and breakfast we were staying at. Then, we headed out to meet up with the group for dinner. It was my husband, three of his sisters, their husbands, and me. Of all of us, only my husband and the birthday girl are reserved. The rest of us are very outgoing—particularly if alcohol is involved.

We walked over to the restaurant and were greeted by the birthday girl's husband. "You'll want to put your drink order in now."

"Why? Do we have some catching up to do?" my husband asked.

"No, they're very slow here."

We walked into a practically deserted restaurant except for our large table at the back of the room, a table for two right next to us, a group of four at the bar, and a collection of dirty dishes on top of every unoccupied table. I surveyed the space, asking, "Do we maybe want to go someplace else?"

The birthday girl decided we should stay. We took our seats as the waitress was getting another round of drink orders for the table. My husband and I jumped in with our orders.

My husband's oldest sister spoke up. "Make it two for them." I looked at her wide-eyed. "Don't worry. They won't show up at the same time, and I bet you one of them shows up after dinner. If you know what you want to eat, you should order that right now, too—trust me."

My husband and I quickly decided what we wanted to eat and tagged that onto the group order. His oldest sister was absolutely right about everything that would happen. My first drink came out in a reasonable amount of time. We sat, drank, and laughed. Our server didn't come back until she had our food, which was about forty minutes after my husband and I ordered (which made it about an hour after the rest of the table had ordered).

Finally, our food came out. Some of us had edible meals; some of us did not. Those with edible food shared with the others, but it still left half the table with mostly alcoholic drinks in their empty bellies.

When we finished dinner, we made our way around the town to various bars. We were about ready to wrap it up for the evening and were discussing what to do the next morning when a total stranger popped her head out of a bar.

"Hey, are you the group from the restaurant up the street?"

We looked at each other. "Yes, yes we are," one of us answered.

"Well, you should come in here!" called the stranger.

We went into this old bar and headed right for the jukebox. What made her recognize us, I wondered? Was it our loud voices, the size of our group? Maybe it was my neck brace. I bet people don't see a middle-aged gal in a neck brace enjoying mixed drinks very often.

My husband and I headed out a little bit after the birthday girl and her husband had left. We returned to the bed and breakfast, had some make-out time, then went to bed. In the middle of the night, I heard this scratching noise.

Those mice! Damnit, this place had mice, too. I hopped out of bed and started knocking on the walls, trying to get the noise to stop. Like a mad woman, I was wandering around this bedroom tapping on walls.

Finally, my husband burst out laughing. "It's the ceiling fan. The ceiling fan is squeaky. Turn off the fan and come back to bed."

I was still too tipsy to be embarrassed.

September 16, 2017

After sleeping in a luxurious amount (probably until 8 a.m.), my husband and I got up and ate some breakfast scones that our bed and breakfast provided. Then, we decided to go out and eat a more substantial breakfast.

When we came back from breakfast, nobody else was up, so we went to work. My husband worked on schoolwork, and I applied for a writing job before working on my website. Finally, we started getting group texts, indicating that everyone was awake and about ready to head out for the day.

We drove around to a couple of nearby wineries and tried some samples. By dinnertime, we all decided that we wanted to eat at a restaurant where everyone would have edible food. We chose correctly, had a great dinner, and went out for drinks.

We stopped in a bar that we hadn't been to before. The waiter said that he had had a broken neck. He ended up with two broken vertebrae and needed surgery, so he has a four-vertebrae fusion. Amazing. Once again, I am so thankful that my break didn't require surgery and that it was as limited and small as it was.

After drinks, we walked around downtown and decided to go to bed early. Most of us were in bed before 10 p.m.

September 17, 2017

When everyone woke up and wanted to meet for breakfast, my husband and I suggested this great breakfast place that we had eaten at the day before. All of us headed over for the last gathering before we would disburse and return to our regular lives.

I was trying to decide what to order today, and the restaurant owner came over to me. Her daughter, one of the cooks, broke her neck, and we were wearing the same neck brace. After I ordered, she took me over to the order window and called over her daughter.

The woman was probably about ten years younger than me. We talked a little bit about how we broke our necks and how uncomfortable neck braces were. Then, I took my seat.

It's crazy. Aside from one guy in high school, I can't remember ever seeing anyone with a broken neck. Now, I'm running into people everywhere I go.

My Pre- and Post-Walk Stretching Routine

26

September 18, 2017

I am so excited to get back to yoga. My entire body needs to stretch, tone, and condition. Please, please, please let me be released from the neck brace on September 27.

After much thought and consideration, I've decided to create an exercise routine combining Pilates and yoga. It's not much, but it shouldn't injure me in the next two weeks until I am (hopefully) released from my neck brace.

NOTE: Before I give you the details about what exactly I did, I want to remind you that I'm not a medical professional, and technically, everything that I'm about to describe doing was against my doctor's orders. I greatly respect doctors, their knowledge, and their advice. However, for me, I felt like adding a little bit of strengthening and stretching would greatly improve how I felt.

Before the Walk

If you would like more information about these and other Pilates exercises and yoga poses, visit my website, www.custompilatesandyoga.com. Here are the exercises that I'm doing along with pictures of me practicing them:

1. Correct neutral alignment

Before you begin walking, use the 5 Basic Principles of Pilates to help you find correct neutral alignment. This will help prevent you from injuring your spine in the future.

The 5 Basic Principles are:

1. Breathing,
2. Neutral pelvis,
3. Neutral rib cage placement,
4. Neutral scapula placement, and
5. Neutral head and cervical spine placement.

Naturally, your neck brace will take care of your neutral head and cervical spine placement. Do your best to get the rest of your body aligned as you practice breathing.

2. Pilates breathing

When we practice breathing, it is an excellent way to prepare for the exercises or activity to come. We inhale to expand the rib cage (particularly in the sides and back, which can be quite closed off), and we exhale to help engage the transverse abdominis and intercostal muscles of the ribs. The intercostals connect the ribs to each other. Specifically, they let the ribs move away from and closer to each other. *This means that the rib cage, as a structure, is supposed to change shape.*

As you inhale through the nose and exhale through pursed lips, think about the benefits you are receiving just from breathing.

- You are oxygenating your blood.
- Focused breathing helps you relax.
- The concentration on your breath helps deepen your body/mind connection.

- The exhale helps to activate the transversus abdominis, your deepest abdominal muscle that is responsible for holding your internal organs in your body cavity.

3. Leg slides

- Begin on your back with your knees bent, heels in line with your SITs bones. SITs stands for Sacral Ischial Tuberosities, but people who don't know that still call them the SITs bones because they're the bones you feel when you sit cross-legged.
- Relax your shoulders away from your ears.
- Make sure your spine is in neutral. If your abdominals are weak, make a triangle with your hands by connecting your pointer fingers and thumbs. Place this under your sacrum (tailbone) to help keep your pelvis neutral throughout the exercise. Otherwise, let your arms rest by your side.
- Take a nice deep inhale.
- Completely exhale. Feel the air leave your abdominal cavity and chest, but don't let your spine move.

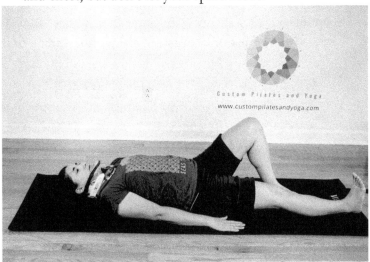

Custom Pilates and Yoga
www.custompilatesandyoga.com

- Inhale and slide your right leg away from you, keeping your heel in line with your SITs bone. You should use your whole inhale as your leg slides away. Flex your foot and feel like a rubber band is connected from your heel to your SITs bone. As your leg straightens, the tension in the rubber band increases.

- When your leg is perfectly straight, immediately exhale through pursed lips and start to bend your knee. Feel the tension in the imaginary rubber band decrease as you draw your heel toward your SITs bone.

- Each time your leg slides, feel your organs settle and your abdominal cavity hollow.

- Do 5-10 reps.

- Switch legs.

4. Leg lift

- Set up the same way you would for Leg slides with your heels in line with your SITs bones, shoulders away from your ears, and arms by your sides.

- While keeping the muscles active that connect your ribs to your hips, inhale into the sides of your ribs. I think of trying to close any space between my armpits and my ribs.

- As you exhale through pursed lips, lift one leg so that the knee is directly over the hip and the ankle is in line with the knee. Choose to do your weaker leg first. This will help you establish a reasonable goal for the number of repetitions on each side.

- Either flex, point, or floint your foot at the ankle. (When you floint, your foot looks like it's wearing an invisible

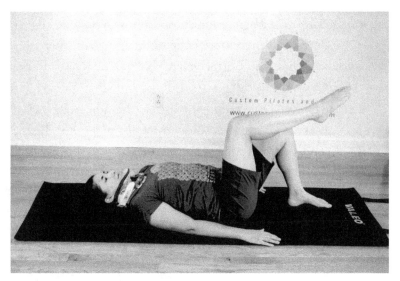

high-heeled shoe. This is a great option for those who get foot cramps.)

- Inhale as you hinge your lifted leg away from you. If you feel your pelvis start to move, you've gone too far.

- Exhale to bring your leg back so that your knee is aligned directly above your hip.

- Do 5-10 repetitions on this side.

- When you are finished, lower the foot to the floor. As the muscles in your working leg relax, you should notice that your pelvis does not rock back to center. (This means it should have stayed centered the whole time.)

- Do the other side.

5. Hip release

- Get set up the same way you would for Leg slides with your heels in line with your SITs bones, shoulders away from your ears, and arms by your sides.

- Before you begin, think about how you're using your abdominals to connect your rib cage to your pelvis. The whole time you do this exercise, your rib cage and pelvis should stay stable.

- Inhale, and open your right knee to the side. Make sure that you use your muscles to open the leg in a controlled way. Keep the lateral rotation of your leg as you slide it until it's straight.

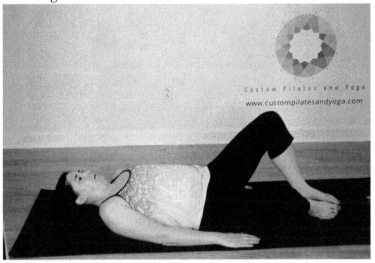

Custom Pilates and Yoga
www.custompilatesandyoga.com

- Exhale, and rotate your leg to parallel. Bend your knee to return to starting position.

- Do 3 repetitions this way; then reverse the sequence.

- Inhale, and slide your leg out straight. Laterally rotate it so that your kneecap faces out to the side. Don't work too hard to do this. It should feel like a nice, natural rotation from the hip.

- Okay, this is a tricky part so pay close attention to your body. Exhale, and bend your knee, still staying open at the hip. As your knee bends, let it move on an upward angle away from your body. This will help your heel stay in line with your SITs bone. If you try to force things or if you don't let your knee come up high enough, your heel will end up in the wrong place. From the hip, return your bent leg back to starting position.

- Do 3 repetitions this way; then switch sides. Make sure to do both directions on your second side.

6. Windshield-wiper legs

- Begin on your back with your feet to the outside edges of your mat.
- Slightly turn out your feet.
- Broaden your collarbones and reach your arms straight out like a "t." Slide your shoulder blades down your back as you bend your elbows and rest the backs of your hands on the mat. This arm pose is frequently called *Cactus*.

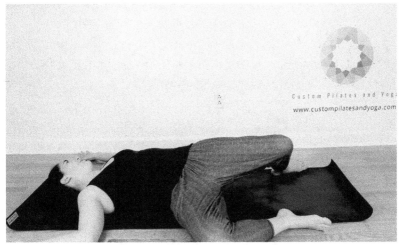

Custom Pilates and Yoga
www.custompilatesandyoga.com

- Let both knees gently lower to the right. Although you might normally allow your head to look to the left, you should not do this cervical movement if you are wearing a neck brace.

- Come back to center.
- Lower your knees to the left.
- Come back to center.
- Do several sets of this at whatever speed and with whatever breathing style feels right.

After the Walk
After walking or whenever I feel like I need some stretching, I practice these 5 poses.

1. Staff Pose (Dandasana)
- Sit on your bottom with your legs straight out in front of you. If it feels like your pelvis is tucked under you, get a blanket (or two) to sit on and rotate your pelvis so you can feel your SITs bones press into the prop beneath you.
- When you feel your low back, you should be able to feel the neutral curve of your spine. It should not be flattened. If it is, grab a blanket to sit on.
- Cross your hands at the wrist and rotate your femurs (thigh bones) in toward your midline. This is called internal rotation. When you do that, you should feel your SITs bones spread and press into the mat. If you do not feel this, gently rock from side to side and use your hand to scoot the muscle tissue near your bottom out to the side. Try again to feel your SITs bones connect to the ground.
- The adductors (inner thighs) work to keep your legs together and in parallel.

- Press the backs of your heels down into the mat as the toes curl back toward you. This should create a wonderful muscular energy like your legs are reaching for the wall in front of them.
- Take your thumbs and press them in to the hip flexors in the fronts of your hips. They should feel soft. If they are active and pressing back in to your thumbs, work on your mind/body connection and ask them to soften. It's okay to work on this for a while. Having soft hip flexors during this posture is very helpful.

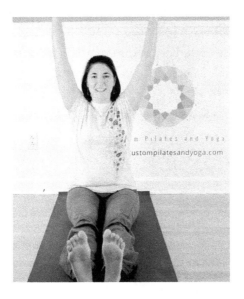

- Now, send energy down through the SITs bones and feel yourself lift toward the ceiling. Feel an energetic lift through the top of your head and align your skull with your spine and pelvis.

- You can leave your arms by your sides or you can lift your arms toward the ceiling with your palms facing each other. I prefer to have my arms lifted because I feel like it helps me lift away from my hips. This feeling of creating more space between my ribs and hips helps to soften my iliopsoas (the main hip-flexing muscle) and build core strength.

2. Seated Forward Fold Pose (Paschimottanasana)

- While you practice this pose, inhale and exhale through your nose. Unless you're congested, you should keep your mouth closed while you breathe.

- Begin seated in Staff Pose. Make sure your femurs are medially rotated (toward the center of the body) and you can feel your SITs bones pressing firmly into the ground.

- Lift out of your hips and allow your pelvis to hinge forward. Keep a straight spine while you let your pelvis hinge. *If you are still in a neck brace, do not allow your head to lower.*

- Place your hands on your calves, ankles, or feet. If this feels uncomfortable, place your hands beside you. Wherever you place your hands, make sure that you are not grabbing anything because grabbing will cause injury.

- As you inhale, think of lengthening the spine and allowing the pelvis to rotate further. On your exhale, think of softening into this pose. Remember, to keep your head lifted if you're in a neck brace.

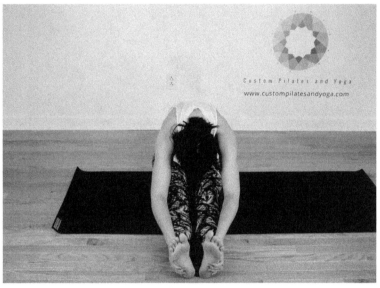

Custom Pilates and Yoga
www.custompilatesandyoga.com

- To create a nice traction for your legs, think of pressing your SITs bones down and back while you reach away with your heels.
- Hold for 8 breaths.
- On your last exhale, draw the belly button to the spine, lengthen, and come up to your starting position.

3. Bound Angle Pose (Baddha Konasana)
- While you practice this pose, inhale and exhale through your nose. Unless you're congested, you should keep your mouth closed while you breathe.
- Begin seated in Staff Pose.
- Bend your knees and allow them to open to the side.

- Bring the soles of your feet together. Make sure that you still feel your SITs bones pressing into the mat. Also, ensure that your right and left foot are pressing evenly into each other.

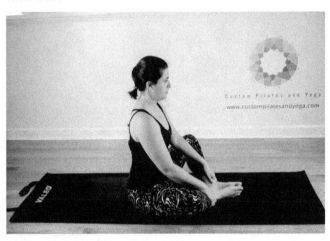

- Allow your heels to come toward your crotch. As your feet move, make sure to keep contact between the right and left foot.
- If your knees are higher than your hips, you can sit up on a bolster or increase the distance between your heels and crotch. Do what you can to bring your hips higher than your knees.
- Use your pointer finger and thumb to loop around each foot's big toe.
- Lengthen through the spine, lifting the ribs away from the hips and drawing the belly button to the spine.
- Hinge from the hips to lower the upper body forward. Keep a straight spine. Be aware that, in order for your spine to move forward, your pelvis must rotate. As the pelvis

moves, so will your SITs bones. *If you are wearing a neck brace, make sure that your head does not lower beneath your heart.*

- Take 5-8 long breaths.
- Engage the abdominals and lift up. You can repeat this or just practice it once.

4. Hero's Pose (Virasana)

- Move onto your hands and knees, bring your knees together, and separate your feet so that they are wider than your hips. The goal here is that you will be able to have so much space between your feet that you could sit on the floor with your feet on either side of your hips.
- Lift your hands off the floor and cross your hands at the wrists. Use your hands to internally rotate your thighs.
- Grab a bolster, block, or blanket (common yoga props) if you think you might need it; and rotate your pelvis so your SITs bones are pointing out and there is a nice curve in your lumbar spine.
- Sit back onto your prop or the floor.
- Feel your SITs bones press down into the floor or prop beneath them. As you feel that connection between your SITs bones and whatever is beneath them, feel how the energy goes up through the crown of your head, giving you a nice long spine.

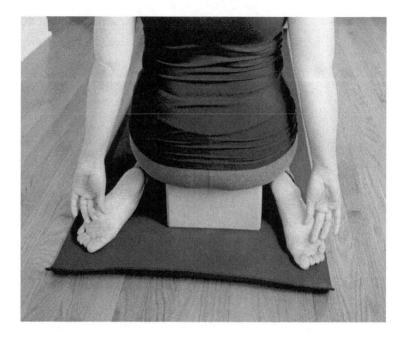

- Broaden the collarbones.
- Make sure your head is aligned with your spine and your chin is not sticking forward.
- I like to take my thumbs and massage my feet while I sit here. You should hold for at least 8 long, slow breaths, so it's nice to give your body a treat to help you be able to stay positive while you practice this challenging pose.

5. Windshield-wiper legs

This is the last exercise in the warm-up, and I like to use it as the last exercise in my cool-down. See page 163 for the instructions and accompanying picture.

Life Without My Neck Brace

27

October 5, 2017

L ast week, I saw my neurosurgeon (hopefully, for the last time). He told me I was free to start living life without my neck brace. When he told me to take my neck brace off, I was confused. Honestly, it's been so long that I thought he was messing with me.

He told me to taper off wearing my neck brace over the next two weeks, so I thought it was kind of crazy to start my life without my brace in his office. I had plans that day: driving, a haircut (the first in many months), and some at-home facial time. I sure didn't want to use up my brace-free time in his office.

The First Day

I discovered that the first day out of the neck brace wasn't that bad. Surprisingly, I worked, drove, had my haircut, and did my facial all without the neck brace. In between events, I put it on and rested.

I think part of the reason I did so well the first day was because I had actually been practicing using my neck muscles for quite some time. When I first broke my neck, the doctor told me I shouldn't wear my neck brace too tightly. Sometimes, when I was feeling good, I would work on holding my head straight and level, centering my neck perfectly in the middle of my collar.

For short periods of time, I would work my neck muscles this way. Then, I would reach up and slide my collar back so my chin comfortably rested on its perch. Once supported, I relaxed my neck muscles and let my collar support me fully.

Rainy Days

For the first couple days, I had great success. Then, around day four, it rained. What a curse! Before the rain had actually started, my neck hurt, and I had a diagonal pain through the right side of my face, passing behind my right eye, up to my scar in my eyebrow.

Anyone with broken bones and arthritis know what I'm talking about. The pain is so sharp and intense that it's like I had re-injured myself. I spent most of my waking hours back in my neck brace.

Honestly, I was hesitant to spend so much time back in the brace after I had been spending most of my waking hours out of it. However, I was pleasantly surprised when I woke up the next morning. I was rewarded with more mobility, greater ease with head movements, and no more pain.

"You Must Be So Happy to Have that Off!"

People always say, "You must be so happy to have that off!" The truth is: I'm not. You see, I somehow managed to escape from a very serious situation with only minor amounts of pain and discomfort. Lots of people who break their necks die, and that fact isn't lost on me.

The neck brace makes sure that, should anything else happen to me in this crazy life, my already-broken neck isn't vulnerable to further injury. All it would take is the wrong kind of bump and I could be in pain, paralyzed, or dead. I don't like any of those options, so I always valued my time with my neck brace.

Now, though, I'm supposed to move on. My neck is showing signs of healing, but the doctor said the indications of healing are not quite as advanced as he would have imagined. He ordered X-rays to make sure my vertebra moved like it should, then gave me the go-ahead.

Now, I feel like I'm living my whole life on eggshells. Don't move too quickly or suddenly. Make sure your head is always level and your shoulders are relaxed. Don't turn your head too far, but don't ignore those muscles that need to be strengthened. The whole thing feels like chaos—chaos with potentially fatal consequences.

What Are You Doing?

I suppose I'm doing pretty much the same things that I did with my collar on.

- Eat healthy foods.
- Walk and stretch.
- Get plenty of sleep.
- Make good decisions.
- Keep my head in neutral and my shoulders away from my ears.
- When I move, I think about the muscles that I need to be using. Then, I try to correctly use those muscles.
- Take deep breaths and remember that this, too, is a process.
- Only move in ways that feel good.
- If I think I might need the brace, I put it on.

I'm so curious to learn what life will be like once I'm fully healed.

What I Missed Most About Yoga Will Surprise You

28

October 21, 2017

I have this issue. It's common and many people have it, but it's my issue and I accept responsibility for it. When I start to fall asleep, if my husband falls asleep first and I can hear him breathe, it drives me bonkers.

I nudge him and roll him; I do whatever I can think of so that I can't hear him. When I put in earplugs appropriate for a shooting range, I still hone in on his sound, and it infuriates me.

Mind you, he's not even snoring. He's breathing, existing peacefully, but the sound of it drives me crazy and keeps me awake.

What I Missed Most About Yoga

When I first started practicing yoga, I had the same issues. We would get ready for Resting Pose (Savasana). Undoubtedly, someone would drift off, and it would rock my boat.

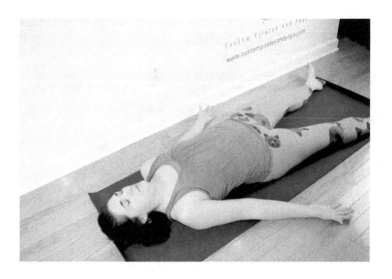

However, since I was approaching this unnerving situation immediately following a wonderful yoga practice, I was able to have a moment of clarity. Instead of being frustrated by the external sound, I should look for the silence within.

When you look at the root of everything, my issue isn't about the noise that someone else makes. After all, the person is breathing. This means that they are healthy and alive. You know what would be quite unnerving? Someone not breathing, because then they'd be dead. That would be terrible.

I may blame this or that external noise (and sure, some noises are going to be more annoying to you than others), but the real problem is within. So, I decided to lean in to the discomfort I felt from listening to the breathing noise. I had to actively relax my shoulders, neck, and jaw constantly in the beginning. Then, one day, without realizing it, I was over it. I had practiced enough that I could create quiet within myself, no matter what was going on around me.

Naturally, I took that skill to the bedroom. My newfound ability to create quiet within me allowed for everyone to have a more restful night's sleep.

With my broken neck taking me away from my physical yoga practice, I became rusty. My old nudging and rolling habits returned until finally, I had had enough. I was sick of the anger, frustration, and blame game.

I decided to ignore my doctor's advice and resume my yoga practice. Resting Pose was the only pose I started practicing, but boy did *that one pose* make a great difference in my happiness.

In Hindsight

I wish I would have been a little less literal with my doctor's orders from the beginning. Yes, I absolutely needed to let my body heal and rest. However, my mind and spirit suffered from the complete removal of my yoga practice.

When you're healing from an injury, you can still practice Resting Pose. You can still feel yourself connect to the ground beneath you and practice breathing. If you have never given meditation a try, it's a great opportunity when you have restricted movement.

Do your best to nurture your spirit when your body is recovering, and your recovery will be more tolerable.

My Self-Rehabilitation Process

29

November 26, 2017

Entertainer Tom Petty told us in a song, "The waiting is the hardest part." Through the years, I've found that to be true during so many different stages of my life. Although I'm certain he wasn't singing about the cervical rehabilitation process, I suppose I could be wrong because waiting has *definitely* been the hardest part for me.

These past two months without my neck brace have been so difficult for two reasons. First, the actual process of creating and attempting to correctly execute my own rehabilitation exercises feels like a daily exercise in futility. Second, with no neck brace, I constantly have a nagging neck pain. This makes the recovery process far worse than any other phase.

Even when I first broke my neck, I slept better than I do now. Without the support of the neck brace, I wake up in pain every hour or two. When I take a full dose of acetaminophen, it keeps me asleep for only about four hours. However, I have experimented and have some tips to help your cervical rehabilitation process go smoothly.

Tips for Cervical Rehabilitation

- **Variety is the spice of life.** Change out the exercises you do. Make sure to work your head so it moves in all directions. Remember, you don't simply need to look left, right, up, and down. You also need to have movement in the in-between areas like up and to the left.

- **Have a team.** You shouldn't do this alone. If you have someone who can make sure you're exercising your neck correctly, use him or her.

- **Try different forms of therapy.** This directly pertains to #1 and #2. I highly recommend that you get acupuncture and have short massages. I know that 15-minute massages have worked well for me. Start with a short time, and you can build from there.

- **Prepare for bedtime.** It may be odd, but I recommend that you build a pillow fort of sorts around your head. Or, I suppose you could buy one of those pillows with a deep divot in the middle and appropriate cervical support. In any case, get yourself fully prepared for bedtime before you start to drift off to sleep.

The Trouble with Sleeping

When you're sleeping (or trying to sleep) is probably going to be the most painful time in your day. What happens is, as your body relaxes, your head starts to drift to one side. Because of your time in your neck brace, your neck muscles are both tight and weak.

Therefore, as your head drifts to the side, it feels okay for a short time. Unfortunately, about the time you start to drift off, you will be hit with an intense pain and the inability to comfortably bring your head back to center. Once the pain begins, your neck is indicating it's already overstretched. This means that the muscle has absolutely no interest in helping you move back to center.

So, you have to use your hands to move your head. The process begins again. You start to drift off, your head rolls to the side, and then you wake up to pain. It's a frustrating cycle that will keep going unless you make a wise change—pillows.

It is worth it to spend some time setting up before you actually go to sleep. If you're a side sleeper, check out your position. Are your head and neck supported enough so you're right up on your shoulder socket? If you sometimes also sleep on your back, what are you going to do? Is there a spot on your pillow that is flat enough to offer the appropriate amount of cervical support?

Take the time to prepare before you turn out the light at night, and you'll have a much better night's sleep. With proper support, your neck will not be in quite so much pain. Plus, if you get a decent amount of quality sleep, you will feel better in the morning.

Learn from my mistakes. I hope that this advice helps you and leads you down a smooth road of recovery.

Alternative Healing Therapies

30

Acupuncture

When I was released from my cervical collar, my doctor didn't prescribe physical therapy as part of my recovery. Instead, he told me that I should be able to do everything myself. Furthermore, he informed me that if I came back complaining of pain, he was going to refer me to a pain specialist.

Needless to say, when I discovered that this time without my neck brace was more painful than any other phase of this process, I did not call my doctor. Instead, I took matters into my own hands.

What To Do

December 2016, my mom discovered acupuncture. She was searching for a therapy to help her continue to improve from the stroke she had several years ago. All the information she read indicated that acupuncture *might* help.

She started receiving regular acupuncture treatments and has noticed significant improvements in several areas affected by her stroke. If acupuncture could help reduce my mom's pain and improve her muscle function, surely it could help me, too.

My Goals

I had two pain-management goals: 1) To be able to turn my head without arresting pain during the day, and 2) To sleep without acetaminophen to dull the constant pain at night. These sounded like reasonable, attainable goals to me, but they were elusive.

No matter how often I stretched my neck and strengthened the muscles, my head would only turn to a certain spot before a spasm of pain stopped my rotation. At night, as I would fall asleep, my head would slightly turn. Right as I'd fall asleep, a muscle spasm would jerk me awake. I was ready for this horrible cycle to be over.

Acupuncture for the Cervical Spine

Luckily for me, my chiropractor also performs acupuncture. I made an appointment and was cautiously optimistic about the results. Previously, she performed acupuncture on me when I was trying to prevent a sinus infection. After the acupuncture treatment, I felt that my sinuses drained and my condition improved. I was hoping she would be able to do something similar for the pain in my neck.

My Treatment

She had me lie down on my stomach and placed needles at several points on my neck and head, at a couple of spots on the back of my legs, and one on the sole of each foot. Most of the time when the needles were inserted, it didn't hurt.

A couple of times, though, it really did. When those spots were hit with the needle, it seemed like a light bulb exploded in my brain. Truly, I believe I saw a flash of light. It was intense and painful but only for a second or two. Then, it was fine.

After she had all the needles placed, my chiropractor left the room to let me rest. At first, I was very comfortable and started to relax into the face cradle. However, after several minutes, my sinuses began to get stuffy and my nose started to clog.

I decided to lift my head to get a temporary break for my sinuses. When I lifted my head, my sinuses opened, but a sharp jolt went from one of the needles in my neck to my brain. Again, another flash of light. I lowered my head as quickly and carefully as I could.

I rested with my head lowered for the rest of the time. Maybe lifting my head and feeling that intense sensation was good, but I didn't want to risk doing damage to myself. After all, if she wanted me to occasionally lift my head, she would have said so.

My Results

I could not have been more pleased with the results from this treatment. Immediately, there was no more pain when I rotated my head. At night, I noticed an improved quality of sleep and was able to make it through the night without acetaminophen. Truthfully, I'm not exactly sure how long the effects lasted because after several pain-free days, I scheduled another session for the following week. My plan is to continue acupuncture weekly in conjunction with the stretches and strengthening exercises that I'm doing for my neck at home.

However, since my acupuncturist is also my chiropractor, she was able to prescribe physical therapy for me. I'm holding onto that script right now like a Wonka golden ticket. If my neck isn't working exactly like it should by January, I'm going to *finally* get to start physical therapy.

Physical Therapy—My First Session

When the new year rolled around, I researched the local physical therapists and ended up selecting the one that my acupuncturist/chiropractor recommended. I chose this office because they perform dry needling. My acupuncturist believes that because acupuncture has worked for me in the past, dry needling will also be helpful.

I was so excited. Finally, after three months of feeling like I was going nowhere, I was going to get the help I needed.

My Assessment

I'm not sure if you've actually thought about the impact of immobilization and the extent of the impact on your body. I *thought* that I had, but I didn't truly understand until I went to physical therapy.

Naturally, the muscles in the neck and shoulders are significantly weakened. Then, I learned very quickly that the entire spine and core muscles are also greatly impacted. I hadn't anticipated this, but the discovery seemed logical.

What I hadn't realized was that the neck brace made it so that I had almost no movement at C6 and T1, and C7 literally had no movement at all. C7 is such an important transition point for your spine. When it locks down, it greatly impacts the ability of other vertebrae up and down the chain to work correctly.

Because of this lock-down, my thoracic vertebrae were unable to help my cervical spine with rotation and other movement. This caused neck pain.

When I would look side-to-side, my head would stop at a point that caused me such intense pain that I couldn't move any further. I had a different experience looking up and down and moving my ear to my shoulder. With those exercises, my head moved as far as it could and then stopped. I had no pain with any of these exercises like when I looked side-to-side.

Get Rid of Pain

The first order of business was to get rid of pain. This was accomplished by loosening tight muscles and encouraging correct movement patterns.

I won't lie—I was extremely pleased that some of the exercises they gave me looked exactly like the Pilates exercises I would do with my clients. Although these exercises were familiar, they were not exercises I was already doing at home myself.

1. Spinal rotation

- Begin in a neutral side-lying position with your shoulder directly under you. Reach your arms straight in front of you. If you are correctly aligned, your fingertips should be even. Your knees should be bent to ninety-degree angles, so your knees are in line with your hips and your ankles.
- Inhale through your nose and lift your top arm toward the ceiling, moving only from the shoulder. Look at your hand as it rises.
- Exhale through pursed lips and rotate your spine by letting your rib cage open toward the ceiling. Keep looking at your hand as your spine rotates. Try to keep your knees close together.

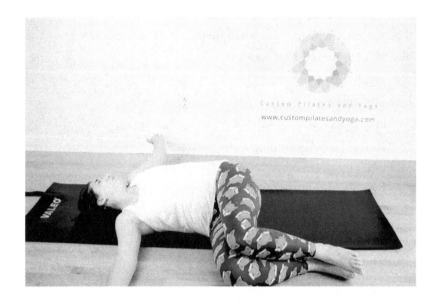

- Hold here for a couple of breaths. As you breathe, tight muscles should relax and you might feel a pop or two in your spine.

- To come out of this rotation, inhale and rotate your rib cage back to neutral. Your top arm should be sticking straight up toward the ceiling.

- Exhale and lower your top hand to meet the bottom hand. If you have come back to neutral position, your fingertips will align.

- You can do as many of these as you want, but I normally only do 2 or 3 on each side. Also, feel free to hold and breathe so any tight muscles you might have can loosen up.

- Switch sides.

2. Cat/Cow Poses

Cat Pose and Cow Pose are both yoga poses. For therapy, my emphasis needed to be on making the most of my spinal flexion and extension.

- Begin on your hands and knees with your hands under your shoulders, fingers spread, and knees under your hips. Draw the low abdominals up toward the spine to support the lumbar spine (low back). Make sure that the scapulas (shoulder blades) are resting flat on the back of the rib cage. Rotate the pelvis out like you are sticking your butt out to the wall behind you. Find the length through your spine to help you reach from your pelvis through the crown of your head. This position is called Table top.

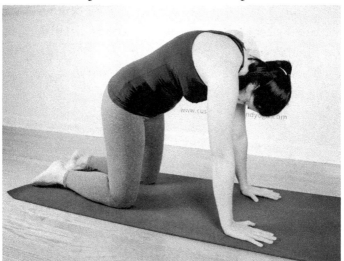

- For this next step, your goal is to achieve an arched spine while you exhale. There are a few ways to accomplish this. You can tuck your pelvis and roll up one vertebra at a time, with your head coming up last. Or, you could drop your head first, and roll up one vertebra at a time, with your tailbone tuck being the last movement. However, you could also drop your head and tuck the tailbone at the same time, sequentially rolling until the middle of your spine reaches up to the ceiling as your apex. There's no wrong way to move through Cat Pose—as long as you are mindful of your movement. *Use your whole exhale to move your body.*

- As you inhale, return to Table top with your hands under your shoulders, knees under your hips, and a nice long spine. Again, you have several choices of how to get to Table top. You could rotate your pelvis back to neutral and move sequentially through your spine until your head reaches to neutral. Or, you could lengthen your head and cervical spine (neck) to neutral, and return one vertebra at a time until the pelvis rotates back to neutral. Also, you could start at the apex of the spine and start lengthening simultaneously toward the head and pelvis. It's up to you. They're all good choices. *Use your whole inhale to lengthen back to Table top.*

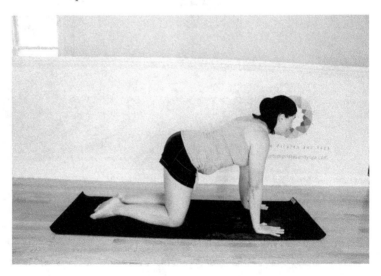

- Inhale to lengthen to a long spine, then allow your heart to rotate forward for Cow Pose. Let your head to lift and your low back arch. Basically, you are doing the complete opposite of the movements that you did for Cat Pose.
- Exhale to lengthen to a long spine then round up to Cat Pose.
- Practice several rounds of this Cat/Cow combination.
- When you are finished, end with a long spine.

3. Thread the needle

Bring your knees wide with your big toes touching, and start lowering your hips toward your heels. Reach your right arm across your chest with your palm facing the ceiling. Slightly rotate your body so your right shoulder touches the ground. Turn your head so your right cheek is also touching. Stretch your left arm overhead with only your fingertips on the mat. Hold and breathe. Then, switch sides.

4. **Look right and left with a soft ball behind your head about 10 times.**
5. **Tuck your chin toward your chest and press the back of your head into a soft ball about 10 times.**
6. **Look up and down with a soft ball behind your head about 10 times.**
7. **Put two lacrosse balls in a pillowcase or sock and use them to massage the occipital part (lower, back part) of your skull.**

These are only a few exercises, but I felt a huge difference after the first therapy session. I practiced my exercises at home over the weekend and, when I returned the following Monday, my pain level was at a 0—as it had been all weekend.

Could This Fix Me?

I'm not sure if I'll ever get my full range of motion back, but physical therapy makes me hopeful. If they can get rid of my persistent skull pain in one session, who knows what else we will accomplish in our time together. Right now, it feels like the sky is the limit for what I can achieve.

Dry Needling

Dry needling is a technique that physical therapists use to relieve pain and tightness. The therapist places a plain needle without medicine, a "dry" needle, through your skin and into a specific area of your muscle.

Normally, the targeted area is a trigger point. For this reason, dry needling is also sometimes referred to as trigger point dry needling (TDN). Trigger points are spots in your muscle that are tight or tender to the touch. In some cases, pressure on one of these points may send pain to another spot in your body.

It's important to note that, while dry needling resembles acupuncture, they are not the same thing. Acupuncture is a part of traditional Chinese medicine, and dry needling is a part of Western medicine. Although they may both have similar goals of releasing tension in a muscle, they have different ways to go about it.

Before You Try Dry Needling

Before you decide to try dry needling, it's important to know that this procedure can be quite uncomfortable and sometimes a little painful. Although the pain is short-term, this treatment is not always a happy, restful experience like acupuncture.

What to Expect

After you've had dry needling, you can expect to feel sore. You may not feel sore immediately, but it may creep in over the next day or so. In order to reduce any soreness you may experience, drink lots of water and take hot baths. Basically, treat yourself like you've had a tough workout at the gym. Or, if you're not familiar with that feeling, treat yourself like you have a cold.

If you have bruises (which happens sometimes), apply ice. Make sure that you don't ice sore muscles since your muscles will probably respond better to heat in this situation.

It's possible that you may feel kind of "loopy" or out of it after your treatment. You may also feel tired, nauseous, emotional, or giggly. All of these feelings are normal and will fade over the next hour or two.

My Dry Needling Experience

I was in physical therapy for a week or two before my therapist agreed that I could try dry needling. We decided to try treating my upper trapezius (a significant neck muscle), which has been a tight and overactive muscle my whole life.

The physical therapist talked to me about all of the feelings and sensations I might experience while she was performing the treatment. She also told me that I might hear a small pinging noise, which would be the needle hitting the base of my skull. When I said I was ready, she began.

All those warnings she gave were no joke. Dry needling was quite uncomfortable. My therapist would stick a needle in a spot, and then move it around. It felt like she was playing spin-the-needle in my neck muscle.

She would move the needle until she found a spot that would make my upper trapezius contract almost to the point that it felt like a muscle cramp. Like I said, this muscle has been overactive on me for a long time, so she didn't have to move very far to find issues.

How I Felt Afterward

I felt terrible afterward. For about 48 hours I felt like I had the flu. I drank water, took warm baths, slept a lot, and tried to massage the muscle. As promised, the pain stopped almost entirely as soon as the 48 hours passed, and I went back to feeling fine.

When I went back for therapy, my regular therapist (a different one from the therapist who performed the treatment) noticed that my head and neck were moving better. I had noticed that the sharp pain that would prevent my head from rotating past a certain point was completely missing. Now, when I looked to the side, my head rotated as far as it could go, and then it stopped.

Would I Recommend It?

It's possible that dry needling is not for everyone. With my situation (where I had constant low-grade pain), I think dry needling was very beneficial. For a fact, it stopped my neck pain that restricted my mobility.

I wasn't sure what this treatment would actually do for me, but the ability to go back to living a pain-free life was worth the gamble. Getting rid of my pain was my main goal, but the increased mobility that I also received was a nice bonus.

If you're thinking about trying dry needling, I recommend that you find a reputable practitioner and talk to that person to find out if you are a good candidate.

IASTM

Instrument Assisted Soft Tissue Mobilization (IASTM) is a rather common component of injury recovery. Some people have described it as a Western version of *gua sha*, the Chinese medicine practice. Although gua sha treats energy along the meridian, IASTM treats musculoskeletal conditions.

The idea behind IASTM is that your trained practitioner applies a forceful massage to your muscle with a scraping tool. This pressure, which causes a microtrauma, can break up fascial adhesions and scar tissue. The pressure from the scraping tool triggers activity inside your body.

Automatically, additional blood is circulated to the area and works to clean out any unnecessary adhesions. Because of this external triggering of your body's cleanup crew, your body can complete the healing process by removing the protective mechanisms of scar tissue and fascial adhesions.

However, there is very little scientific research that substantiates these claims—much like with gua sha. So, although this may work, it isn't scientifically proven as an effective treatment.

Because IASTM is so common, you might be able to find a local physical therapist that practices this technique. The best way to know for sure is to call around. Once you have a list of a couple people who practice this technique, ask your friends to see if anyone has any particular recommendations.

Astym Therapy

Scientists and researchers created Astym therapy. This is extremely unique. Normally, forms of therapy exist and then are tested, which determines whether or not they are effective. With

Astym, the research was done beforehand to create an effective method.

The scientists particularly looked to advancements and discoveries regarding cells and tissue repairs. This helped inform their decision about tool design and therapy protocol.

Astym vs. IASTM

When you look at Astym versus IASTM, there are a few major differences:

1. Scientists created Astym, and IASTM is the Western version of the Chinese practice of gua sha.
2. Because scientists created Astym, quite a bit of research exists that proves its effectiveness in a variety of situations.
3. The scientists behind the Astym system guard their reputation. Because this is a process that has been developed rather recently, Astym is sort of like a brand name of instrument assisted soft tissue mobilization. Practitioners must undergo a specific training and use Astym-approved tools in their practice.
4. Perhaps because of the very specific training, it seems that Astym might be a gentler practice. When I researched IASTM, I saw some pictures and comments indicating that bruising would be normal. I can honestly say that in all the times that I received Astym treatment (which probably totals over 20 times), I have never had a bruise or any sort of pain from treatment.

Although there are differences, Astym and IASTM have some similarities. The main similarity is that they both truly want to accomplish the same thing. Both practices want to break up and remove scar tissue and unnecessary adhesions. They do this by applying pressure with a tool and encourage increased blood flow to the impacted area.

To find an Astym therapist near you, check out the Astym website's provider search (https://www.astym.com/Patients/ProviderSearch).

Once you know of the nearby locations that offer services, call to find out more information. Ask which therapists practice the Astym method and find out about their availability.

If you are fortunate enough to have many therapists to choose from, ask friends if anyone has had any particularly memorable experiences. This input may help you make your final decision about where to go.

My Experience

I love this therapy! Astym is what my physical therapist uses on me, and I have noticed a great difference. I feel like my neck is more relaxed after she works on me, and I have a reduced amount of pain. If you have the opportunity to try this out, I highly recommend it.

Physical Therapy

31

January 18, 2018

Today was another session of physical therapy. Let's say that the session hit a nerve in more than one way. I was doing Spinal rotation, and my tailbone popped. I supposed I said something like, "Well, that's better."

"Why is that?" asked my physical therapy intern.

"Because I popped."

"Oh, where did you pop, Sarah?"

"My sacrum."

"And that feels fine?"

"Things always feels fine when they pop back into place."

Then, the intern and my physical therapist proceeded to tell me all about how the sacrum doesn't *pop* out of place—that if it did *pop* out of place on me, I wouldn't be able to walk. Seriously, they lectured me about my answer.

This is one my very top pet peeves. I firmly believe that no one should tell someone else that his or her feelings are incorrect. Instead, if you ask me a question, I expect you to listen to my answer. I certainly don't expect you to tell me that I'm wrong, particularly if you have asked me a question about my own body and how I feel.

So, as I'm being tag-team lectured, I cannot focus. I have no idea what they're saying because I'm so livid. The only thing I can think is *Make sure you're nodding and say, "Oh, okay" occasionally so that they don't know how upset you are.* I didn't want to cause a scene or prolong this conversation.

I was taking deep breaths and trying to calm my inner rage. While I was breathing, I decided that I wouldn't tell them that multiple chiropractors have realigned my sacrum in the past and have told me that my sacrum was out of place. What is the point talking to people who aren't listening?

The answer is: there is no point. I wished I had realized that before my session progressed, but I didn't.

Next up, I had asked to try dry needling. I was very excited to try this new technique and see if it could help me. This particular therapist came highly recommended as someone who effectively practices this.

I put on my nice face and tried to make small talk while she put me through a form of hell. Afterwards, my muscles felt extremely sore and tight, but that's to be expected.

We finished up with some mobility exercises. As I would rotate to the right, I could feel the muscles along my spine trying to engage and rotate me further. When I rotated to the left, I would try to move, and it felt like the muscles had shut off.

The physical therapy intern asked me if that left side felt like it was a good challenge. To me, that's a stupid question. No, it's not a challenge. It's not working—at all. I gave him a version of that answer (omitting the part about how stupid I thought the question was), and then I was lectured again.

Out of nowhere, the physical therapist jumps in with a fantastic monologue about how the words we say physically impact our bodies. Again, I'm so upset that I'm simply trying to keep a calm exterior demeanor. As I decide that I have my emotions under control, I focus on what she's saying in time to hear some statistic about how negative words will make your recovery 30 percent less effective, and how she's sure that I would want to change my verbiage and say that the muscle was *challenged.*

I almost lost it. If I go to turn on my furnace, which right now is completely dead and won't heat anything, it's not that the furnace is finding heating my house *challenging.* It's that the wires and parts that need to appropriately communicate are not doing that. It's broken.

I smiled politely, gathered my things, and left. Man, I hope I don't have her ever again.

March 22, 2018

Turn On My Muscles—The Next Step in Neck Therapy

The next session was with my regular therapist. I told her that I felt like my left-side neck muscles were absent. "It's not like they're not working. They're not even in the building. Their cubicles are empty, and they're like outside on the longest break ever."

My physical therapist assessed, and I agreed, that it was time to turn on my muscles. As you can imagine, it's not like a switch flips and functionality and movement are restored to your dormant muscles. Several steps must be taken in a certain sequence to get your body where it needs to go.

To continue with my analogy from above, in order to have people working, you have to find them outside the building and convince them to come into the building. Then, you have to talk them into sitting in their cubicle and eventually doing something. (As someone who has worked in a cubicle, I have experienced this analogy with actual people.)

In the beginning of my therapy, we focused on achieving and maintaining my pain relief (which was my top priority). I regularly practiced my assigned exercises. Whenever my head or neck started to hurt, I would use two lacrosse balls in a sock to massage the back edge of my skull.

Although these exercises also increase mobility, I felt like my body was lacking. When I twisted one direction, I could feel the muscles on the right working. However, when I twisted the other way, it was a void from C6-T1. Any rotation that might happen came from another spot.

Therapy

Lucky for me, I have an amazing physical therapist. She started having me work on a foam roller. The first day we tried to turn on my muscles, she had me practice these three Pilates exercises on the foam roller:

1. **Arm scissors**
   - Come onto your back. To get on the foam roller, make sure that you sit all the way at one end of the roller so that, as you lie down, you don't run out of support. Your pelvis, spine, and head should all be supported by the roller. If your head is off the roller, you can either wiggle your way down so that you're fully supported, or you can roll off and try again.
   - Once you are on the roller, press your feet firmly into the floor and use your abdominals to keep you centered.
   - Reach your arms toward the ceiling with your palms facing each other. Make sure to keep your elbows straight throughout this exercise.

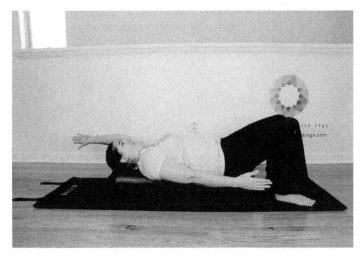

- Inhale through your nose and reach your right arm up by your head as your left arm comes down by your side.
- Exhale through pursed lips and return your arms back to center so they're reaching above your chest.
- Inhale and reach your left arm up by your head as your right arm comes down by your side.
- Exhale and return your arms back to center so they're reaching above your chest.
- Complete 10 sets.

2. **Snow angels**

- Bring your arms to the midline of your body. From the shoulders, rotate your palms toward the ceiling. This may create quite a stretch at the shoulders.

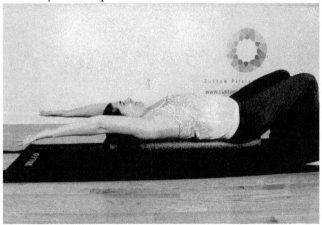

- As you inhale through your nose, sweep your arms by your sides and reach overhead. Make sure that your shoulder blades slide down and to the sides. This movement will help keep your shoulders out of your ears.

- Exhale through pursed lips and bring your arms, palms facing up, back by your sides.

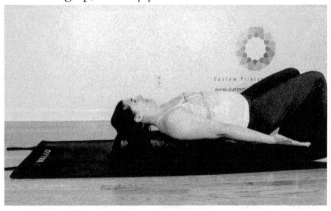

- Do 10 repetitions. Pay particular attention to your shoulder placement throughout this exercise.

3. Hug a tree

- Bring your arms up toward the ceiling with your palms facing each other. Put a soft bend in your elbows so that your fingertips come toward each other and your arms resemble a hoop. Make sure your shoulders are out of your ears and your shoulder blades are in neutral.

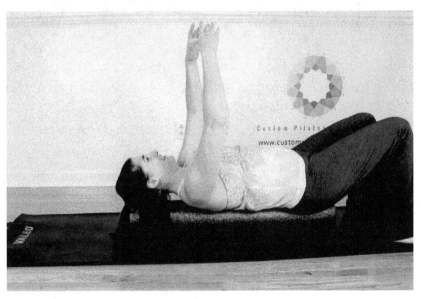

- Keep your arms stable in this position as you move from the shoulders.
- Inhale through your nose to let your arms open to the side.

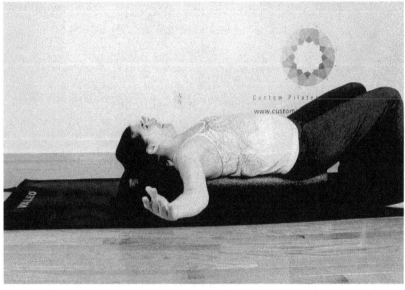

- Exhale through pursed lips to bring your arms back to your starting position.
- Do 10 repetitions. Pay particular attention to your shoulder placement throughout this exercise.

Then, the therapist performed some scraping (which is physical therapy talk for massage with a plastic tool) and moved parts of my spine while I relaxed.

When she finished, she had me do a spinal rotation exercise from the previous week. It was still fresh in my mind how the muscles on my right side worked to rotate while the muscles on my left were nowhere to be found. To my delight, when I went to use the muscles on the left, *they were there.*

To go back to my office analogy, the left-side neck muscles came into the building, made it to their cubicles, and were sitting in a seat. They weren't working quite yet, but they were there. And, for the first time in a long time, I could feel it.

After I left my physical therapist's office, I was so overwhelmed with feelings that I cried. I felt joy and relief because I had been reunited with missing muscles, and I felt pride and accomplishment because my therapist and I did something that I wasn't certain was possible.

Although I had been hopeful that I could reconnect with my missing muscles, I wasn't certain. The relief I felt discovering that we could find my muscles again made me feel like I had just achieved the biggest accomplishment of my life thus far.

April 9, 2018

Respect the Progress

I know that "respecting the process" can be very challenging. In my case, I sat around for about three months wearing a neck brace while waiting for my neck to heal. Then, when the doctor released me from it, I was scared to death to take it off. That shift of thought caused an internal struggle.

The day before I was cleared to take off my collar, it was a life-saving device that was keeping me from death or paralysis. Then, the next day, I was supposed to start wearing it less and less so that I wouldn't use it after a week or two.

That's crazy to be so dependent on something and then turn around and not use it anymore.

However, it's important to understand that while you were healing, your body was preparing you to be less and less dependent on your neck brace. Without knowing it, your body was preparing for this moment. The trick is to get your brain to catch up with your body.

As with anything difficult, take a deep breath and move forward. In this case, it meant taking off my brace. Once I did that, my next hurdle was to start physical therapy.

Where Am I Now?

Since I began physical therapy, I've started to feel my neck change in so many great ways. I have moved fully through the guarded and concerned phase. Now, I sometimes forget that I had broken my neck.

It's the occasional tight muscle or limited movement that keeps me aware that I'm still in the healing process. However, I feel like I'm at a great point in my recovery.

I still feel gains in strength and stability from my exercises and relief from the massages that I receive at physical therapy. I'm doing so well that I have therapy only every other week now. I've come so far. My head turns all the way to the left with only minor strain. It's not quite as nice when I turn to the right, but I know that my range of motion has greatly increased. Similarly, my neck moves like it should when I look down, but it struggles a little when I look up.

Be Grateful

When I look at where I am now, versus where I was a couple months ago, I can't help but be elated. At the beginning of physical therapy, my primary goal was to not be in pain every day. (They fixed that after our first session.) My secondary goal was to regain mobility in my neck, and we're still working on that.

Whenever I'm doing physical therapy (either on my own or at their center), I take a moment to appreciate my advancements. With nothing but hope and gratitude, I move forward and try to strengthen myself. Maybe someday I won't need to take the time and appreciate all the progress that I've made on this journey, but today isn't that day.

Today, I choose gratitude.

May 6, 2018

The End of Physical Therapy

It has happened—after four months of physical therapy, I have been released by my physical therapist, and it feels surreal. A few months ago, I was reliant upon a cervical collar to help keep me from becoming paralyzed or dying. Now, I'm able to do almost everything that I could do before breaking my neck.

How Am I Doing?

You know what? I'm great! After my neck healed and I was released from my neck brace, I was in such constant pain that I started to worry. My main goal was pain relief. Ever since I removed the neck brace, I took several acetaminophens a day to dull the constant, nagging pain—until I started my physical therapy. My very first day in physical therapy, we accomplished my main goal. Since that first session, I've only had some intermittent pain here and there.

My second goal was improved range of motion. Keep in mind that range of motion for your neck isn't simply a left, right, up, down kind of thing. Instead, your head swivels and you have varying degrees of looking up or down and to the sides. This is a real challenge. However, when I practice moving my head in this way, I find great improvement in my range of motion and overall neck mobility.

My Care Plan

Okay, it's true that, like many people post-injury, I do not practice my physical therapy as often as I should. In our last session together, my physical therapist created this beautiful and sometimes intense sequence for me to practice, but I don't always feel like I have a free hour.

Instead, I prefer to practice the yoga sequence that she and I created together. Below, I've described both plans.

Remember, if you think that you have injured your neck, go to your doctor. He or she can order all of the appropriate imaging, medicine, and therapy necessary for you to appropriately heal.

The Bosu Workout

Because I enjoyed using the Bosu ball so much in physical therapy, I decided to buy my own to help improve my balance. This workout is divided into two segments: Bosu ball up and Bosu ball down. When the Bosu ball is up, you can challenge both sides of your body independently. By turning the Bosu over, you can create a sort of wobble board. Either way, you challenge your stability.

Bosu Ball Up

- **Cervical range of motion.** Look right and left about 10 times. Make sure that your head rotates fully. Don't let your chin jut forward. Next, look up and down about 10 times. To look down, tuck your chin toward your neck and roll down one vertebra at a time. Practice the above exercises these three ways: 1) while standing on one leg (in the center of the Bosu), 2) on your hands and knees (with your hands on the Bosu), and 3) kneeling (with your knee on the Bosu instead of the ground). Make sure to do 10 repetitions (reps) for each direction in each position.

- **Lunges.** First, practice side lunges toward the Bosu. Complete 10 reps on one side before switching to the other. Then, place the Bosu in front of you. Lunge to the center of the Bosu, shift your weight, and lift your back leg up so that you're balancing on one leg in the center of the Bosu.
- **Sunbird.** Try this exercise with your hands on the Bosu, and then with your knees on the Bosu. Complete about 10 reps on each side.
  - Begin on your hands and knees with your hands under your shoulders and your knees under your hips. Make sure your fingers are spread.
  - Make sure you use your abdominals to support your low back. Slide your shoulder blades away from your ears.
  - Keeping your abdominal engaged, inhale into the sides of your ribs, and extend your right leg. Flex your foot and keep your toes on the floor.
  - As you exhale, lift your right leg by using your gluteus maximus muscle—the large muscle of your butt. Let your leg lift only as high as you can maintain complete stability with the rest of your body. (Be sure you don't allow your abs to release. This will make your rib cage drop and shoulders slide out of place.) The leg should never lift higher than hip-level.
  - Engage your adductors (inner thighs) to make sure your leg is not drifting or rotated to the side.
  - Inhale and slide your left arm straight in front of your left shoulder with the palm facing the midline of the body.

o   Exhale and lift the arm. Allow the shoulder blade to slide down and out to the side so the arm can lift without the shoulder coming by the ear.

o   Hold here and breathe at least 5 slow breaths.

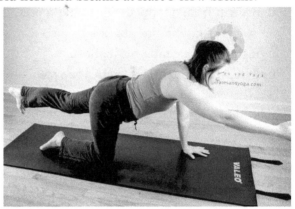

o   Inhale, then exhale and lower the arm and leg at the same time. Allow your fingertips and the tips of your toes to touch the mat; then slide back to starting position.

o   Do the other side.

o   You should do each side at least twice.

Bosu Ball Down

- **Cervical range of motion.** Look right and left for about 10 repetitions. Make sure that your head rotates fully. Don't let your chin jut forward. Next, look up and down for about 10 reps. To look down, tuck your chin toward your neck and roll down one vertebra at a time. Practice these exercises while balancing on one leg (with your foot in the center of the Bosu), with your hands shoulder-width on the flat surface and your legs extended behind you (this is called Plank position), and with your elbows beneath your shoulders and legs extended behind you (in Forearm plank position). Make sure to do 10 reps for each direction in each position.

- **Squats.** Stand with your feet hip-distance apart and parallel on the Bosu. Now, squat as low as you can while keeping your spine straight and your pelvis in neutral. Complete about 10 squats.
- **Bowling statue.** While standing on one leg, let the other leg lift straight behind you. Then, return to upright, bend the leg that was behind, and reach the opposite arm toward the ceiling. Complete about 10 reps on each side.
- **Plank.** Place your hands under your shoulders, straighten your legs, and don't let your hips drop. Plain and simple, hold your best possible Plank at the end of your workout for as long as you can. Shoot for 30 seconds as your goal.

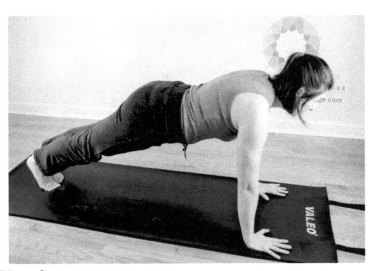

My Yoga Sequence

To get the most out of these poses, you want to practice them in a fluid, sequential way. Notice that you'll practice the poses for the right side then the left. Below are descriptions for how to do these yoga poses along with pictures of me doing the pose.

Here's our sequence:

1. **Downward dog**
   - Let's first take a moment to appreciate that the shape we are creating looks like an upside down "V," not a "U." This means two things: the weight must be evenly distributed between the arms and the legs, and the pelvis *must* be rotated out so that it feels like you're sticking your butt out at the upper part of the wall

   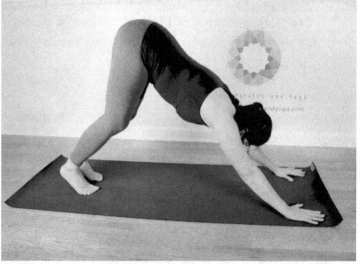

     behind you.
   - Come on to your hands and knees, with your knees hip-width apart. Place your hands at the front of your mat. Spread your fingers like a starfish and create a dome with the middle of your palm. Walk your knees back a little bit, curl your toes under, draw your low

belly to your spine, and lift up like your hips are being lifted toward the ceiling for you.

- Keep a soft bend in the backs of your knees. Let your bent knees free your body to really rotate your pelvis up toward the ceiling. With your feet in this wider, outer hip-width stance, you are able to create openness in the sacrum (tailbone). If you're more comfortable with your legs together or inner-hip distance apart, you're welcome to make that adjustment.

- Lift your chest up slightly and shift your weight forward while keeping the abdominals engaged. Put a slight bend in your elbows. Rotate your arms so that the eyes of your elbows are facing forward. Straighten your arms and move back into position, feeling a broadening sensation across your collarbones and the front of your chest.

- Feel the energy in your arms as you press the floor away from you.

- Notice that your shoulders are very far away from your ears.

- Check that your ears are between your biceps (upper arms).

- As you breathe, think "lengthen on the inhale, soften on the exhale."

- Check your alignment and make any corrections you feel are necessary. If you would like, you can alternate bending your knees to pedal out your feet. When your hamstrings feel warmed up, draw the abdominals to the spine, lift the hips, and lengthen the backs of the legs (be sure not to lock the knees).

2. **Plank pose**

- Hinge forward from the hips so that your shoulders are directly above your wrists.
- Imagine a line of energy from your heels through the top of your head.
- Draw your belly button to your spine to support your lumbar spine (low back). Make sure your low back isn't sagging and that you are not rounding your spine between your shoulder blades.

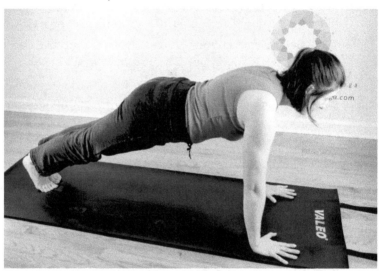

- Keep the abdominals engaged that are connected to your bottom ribs. It can be easy to let those muscles relax, and it ends up pulling on your low back.
- Breathe.

3. **Crescent lunge (right leg back)**
- Step your left leg forward between your hands.

- Your right leg should be reaching back quite a distance so that you have a large space between your right and left feet.

- Make sure that your legs are running parallel to each other, like they are on train tracks but not on the same rail.

- Reach through your right heel like it is reaching for the wall behind you. Take a moment to make sure that your right heel is in a straight line and not rotated in or out.

- Check to make sure that your left knee is in line with the center of your foot. It's okay for the knee to come forward toward the second and third toes, but it should not go past the toes. Also, the knee should not drop toward the inside or the outside of your leg.

- Feel your adductors (inner thighs) reach past each other.

- Draw the low belly to the spine so you can feel yourself lift away from your left thigh without lifting your fingers off the floor.

- As you reach through your right heel, feel yourself reach through your leg, spine, and out through the top of your head. When you find alignment, you can feel energy run through you like a current.

- Draw your belly button to your spine and lift your upper body.

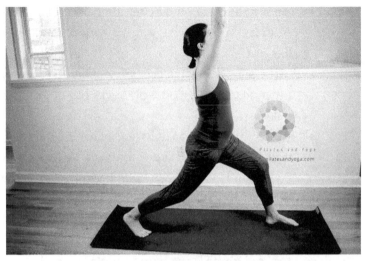

- I like to put my hands on my hips to make sure my pelvis is level and in neutral. Frequently, because of my tightness, it's tilted slightly forward. To correct the tilt of my pelvis, I lift up out of the pose a little bit, bring my pelvis upright, re-engage my core muscles, then lower my pelvis back into the lunge.
- Keeping the core engagement, bring bent arms up so that your elbows are in line with your shoulders and your palms face forward. This is called *Cactus pose.*
- Soften the space in your upper back right behind your heart. As that portion of your upper thoracic spine moves, so will your cervical spine (neck). The head and neck should not drop behind the body but should instead be a natural extension from the thoracic.
- Reach your arms straight toward the ceiling with palms facing each other. Your biceps (upper arms) should be beside your ears. Your hands should be close together, as if you are holding a basketball above your head.
- Hold this side for 5-10 breaths.

4. **Warrior 3 (right leg back)**

- Feel the left foot actively press the floor away, and straighten the left leg.
- Allow the right foot to hop about three inches closer toward the left foot.
- Lift the ribs away from the hips and draw your belly button to your spine. This should not change the placement of your pelvis.

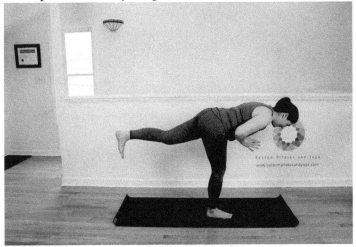

- Think of pushing the floor away from you with your left leg as you lift your ribs away from your hips. Let your upper body hinge forward from the waist. As you do this, your right leg raises behind you.
- Find the adductors (inner thighs) scissor toward each other and make sure your pelvis is not rotated.
- Flex your right foot so that the toes point down to the ground.
- From your right heel through the top of your head is a straight line of energy.

- You don't have to lift your back leg very high. It is more important to feel your supporting leg press the floor away and your abdominals keeping your spine in a straight line.
- Hold for 5-8 breaths.

5. **Tree pose with upper thoracic extension (right leg rotated out)**
    - Let the left leg keep pressing the floor away as you rotate so you're standing upright and balancing on your left leg.
    - Externally rotate your right leg from the hip so your right knee is pointing to the side.
    - Bring the sole of your right foot to your left ankle, left calf muscle, or left thigh muscle.

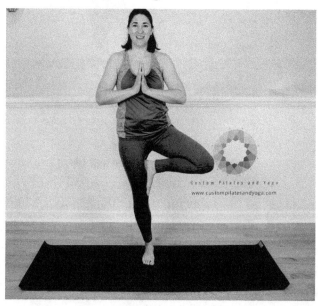

- Send energy from the sole of your right foot to your left leg, from your left leg to the sole of your right foot.

- Place your hands on your hips for a moment to ensure your hips are still facing forward. Sometimes, the hips will drift to the side as the lifting leg rotates open.
- Gently join your palms and bring your hands up to heart center.
- Broaden your collarbones and reach your arms by your ears, straight toward the ceiling.
- Hold here for 5-8 breaths.

6. **Warrior 3 again (right leg back)**
7. **Crescent lunge again (right leg back)**
8. **Plank**
9. **Crescent lunge (left leg back)**
10. **Warrior 3 (left leg back)**
11. **Tree pose with upper thoracic extension (left leg rotated out)**
12. **Warrior 3 again (left leg back)**
13. **Crescent lunge again (left leg back)**
14. **Plank**
15. **Downward facing dog**

It's Been a Year Since I Broke My Neck

32

June 29, 2018

Happy Anniversary! It's been a year since I broke my neck while trying to teach my boys how to play baseball. Although my broken neck was a serious consequence of my fall, it wasn't my only injury. My neck is fully healed, so here's an update about my other injuries from my fall.

My Head and Face

When I head-butted the metal door frame, I hit it so hard that I left a dent in the metal, and pieces of baked-on paint came off onto my hair. After I washed my hair for the first time post-accident, little bits of paint were still stuck in there. It took days for the paint to fully come out.

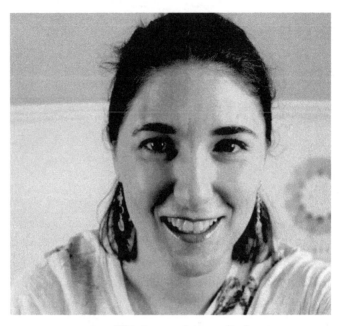

This is me today, unedited.

The impact left me with a dent on the right side of my forehead. It's not terribly noticeable all the time but, when I get in certain light at the right angle, you can clearly see the dent. Also, you might notice that my whole right eyebrow did, in fact, grow back nicely.

My Thigh

When I fell, I banged my left thigh on our wooden back step, which left quite a bruise. This was by far the worst bruise I've ever had. It was amazing to see the different colors that emerged day after day and even week after week.

After about a month, no more bruise was left. In its place was a dent about four-inches long. Despite a valiant attempt to roll the dent out of my leg with The Orb, it is still there.

My Knee

The only injury that even remotely compared to the severity of my broken neck was my right knee. As I was falling and moving at the same time, I drug it across our patio, skinning the whole knee.

This whole time that my neck has been healing, my knee has also been healing. When the wound was fully closed, the nerves in my knee were messed up. It took months before I could allow my right knee to touch the floor. I discovered this the hard way when I accidentally tried to kneel on my right knee to change my son's diaper. The pain was so horrible and intense that I cried immediately and had to take acetaminophen daily for about a week after the incident.

When I could apply pressure to my knee, I started applying special oils to help the discoloration and scarring. Then, after months of being pain-free in my knee, it started intensely hurting again. I started massaging it to break up scar tissue.

Now, here we are at present day. It doesn't hurt and it moves fine, but sometimes my three-year-old forgets and asks, "Oh, Mama! What did you do to your knee?"

"Well, son, this one time I was teaching you and your brother how to play baseball..."

October 30, 2018

The Best Way to Turn Life's Tricks into Treats

You've probably heard that you should use the lemons the life gives you to make lemonade. And while turning tricks into treats is a similar sentiment, not all of life's cruel jokes come off sour like a lemon.

Sometimes, they are *harsher*. More than a bitter taste in your mouth, they can hurt you to the core. Accidents happen. Loved ones die. Then, you're left to pick up the mess like the man behind the elephants at the circus. Bring your shovel.

The challenge and, incidentally the *thing* that will define you, is how you recover from the situation. What you do post-trauma will determine whether or not you can turn your trick into a treat.

Turning Tricks Into Treats

Forrest Gump taught me that life is like a box of chocolates; you never know what you're gonna get. The movie *Parenthood* taught me that life is like a roller coaster and that, although we wish we were on a Merry-Go-Round, we're all still on a roller coaster. And *The Karate Kid* showed me that even when you're down, you're not out.

Yet, with all of the various life lessons that I've learned from movies, nobody has ever taught me how to flip the script and turn a horrible situation into an opportunity. I had to figure that one out on my own.

After My Accident

When the doctor told me my neck was broken and I'd be in a neck brace for around three months, it felt like a knife twisted in my gut. My soul crumpled, and more than my neck felt broken.

I was getting into the groove on my blog. With a commitment to publish a post every day in the first year, I was writing and researching constantly. When I wasn't doing that, I was in front of the camera filming how-to videos for different yoga poses and Pilates exercises. I had no idea how I was going to continue post-accident, but I knew I couldn't continue as usual.

Although my physical pain was managed, I hurt like no other time in my life. Thinking about the list of things I *wouldn't* be doing this summer (driving, swimming, enjoying any social event) was completely overwhelming. Plus, I knew both Pilates and yoga would be out of the question. What the heck was I going to do?

For a moment, I started to entertain the idea that this was it—the end of my blog. Quickly, I decided that wasn't what I wanted. I *wanted* something from this. If I was going to be wearing a neck brace for the hottest months of the year, if I was going to have my harmonious workflow interrupted, I was going to get something.

Trick or Treat—You Decide

Yeah, I was going to get something from this whole horrible experience, and, I decided, it would be wonderful.

I firmly believe that whenever something particularly horrible happens, something mind-blowingly fantastic is around the corner. When you find yourself in the situation where something horrible has happened, ask yourself this one question: *What's in it for me?*

Do This Now!

Decide what you want to learn or receive from your situation and precede with that in mind. In my case, I decided that I wanted to end up with a book about my experience with my broken neck. This decision is the key to flipping your situation and turning your trick into a treat.

When you decide what you want, you are now empowered—pursuing a goal that you created for yourself. However, without that change in perspective, you may feel like a victim, a recipient of misfortune.

The next time you find yourself sucker-punched by life, try to put a spin on your situation and decide what *you* want from your experience. That simple question to yourself may be exactly what you need to flip the script and turn your trick into a treat.

Questions & Answers from Sarah

33

December 13, 2018

Q: When you broke your neck, you had no idea that anything serious was wrong because you had no pain or other indications. What were your first thoughts when they told you your neck was broken?

A: I didn't believe it. I thought it was all some sort of misunderstanding like the guy who read the X-ray results read them incorrectly. Actually, I thought the doctor would come in in the morning and tell me they had misread my results. Then, I started this odd process where I somehow convinced myself that a fracture wasn't a break.

Q: What was your biggest challenge throughout this process?

A: Gosh, where to start? There have been so many challenges, but I think the hardest part was the post-recovery pain. I didn't anticipate that, so I think this is why that particular phase was the most difficult for me.

Q: What was your biggest success?

A: Writing a book. I have never written a book before, but I have always wanted to. For a long time, I felt like I didn't have anything important to say. After breaking my neck, *I had plenty to say.*

Q: Was there anything that you particularly enjoyed? Or loathed?

A: I especially liked the "forced" slow pace. I had become used to doing things quickly. I liked being forced to rest and eat more mindfully. Plus, I loved mentally justifying my nightly ice cream habit—regardless of whether it caused me to gain weight.

As a creature who loves her schedule, I particularly loathed the disruption to my schedule. I had plans, you know? Things to do, vacations to take, afternoons to spend by the pool—then, all of that went down the drain.

Q: How did your broken neck impact you in your work life? Social life? Home life?

A: It changed all of it. My work schedule was completely thrown up in the air, but my broken neck gave me the grit and determination that I would follow through on my goal of one blog post a day for an entire year. You have to take a moment to reflect and figure out how you can work smarter, not harder.

My social life greatly improved. Friends popped by with food or to drive me places. Family members came by regularly to help shuttle me around, which I liked a lot.

What I didn't like is going out in public. I felt like people stared or wanted to ask me questions. It's hard to have someone tell you that you could have died when you're in a kind of fragile emotional state. That's hard to hear, and I think it comes off as insensitive that they would say that, but I know they don't mean to be.

Then, there's this sort of stigma. I felt like I couldn't complain because I was so lucky in so many ways, but at the same time, I sure had plenty of complaints. I was afraid if I told people how uncomfortable I was, they would tell me to be grateful that I hadn't died. Emotionally, I felt like I was in a no-win situation socially.

Of course, my home life changed, too. However, my husband and my boys are total champs. Of the three areas, my home life changed the least—with my husband starting college, my older son starting kindergarten, and my younger son starting preschool.

Q: What will you take from this experience?

A: I feel like the Universe always has a plan. Although you don't understand it, the plan is in motion for greatness. Personally, I hope I can help other people with broken necks. I hope my information helps them be more comfortable with their brace and helps them feel less alone.

Q: How did it feel the first day you were neck-brace free?

A: Terrifying and liberating. I was free to do everything I wanted but unsure if I would still be alive by the end of it all.

Q: What's the first thing you did after you took off your collar?

A: I looked at my doctor and asked him about physical therapy. I'm still so frustrated that I hadn't started physical therapy immediately after he released me from wearing the brace. If your doctor releases you from wearing your neck brace and doesn't prescribe physical therapy, go find someone who will. Physical therapy is essential if you're going to get back to normal.

Q: Have you had a moment yet where you feel like you're back to your old self?

A: Yes! For months now, I feel back to my old self. I can move probably about as well as I could before the break.

Q: What has surprised you most about having a neck brace?

A: I was most surprised by how alone and isolated I felt. When I went out in public, I felt like people stared at me. It made me feel like a walking freak show, and I felt very alone.

Q: When you took off the neck brace, did you put it in the trash or a donation pile immediately?

A: Actually, I have it in my closet right now. I'm still holding out hope that I can dress up as Joan Cusack's character from *Sixteen Candles* for Halloween sometime. Once I find that sweatshirt, I'm in.

Q: What is your favorite part about no longer wearing a neck brace?

A: I would have to say driving is my favorite part. When I can drive, I can go to drive-thrus, and avoiding cooking is one of my favorite pastimes.

Q: I'm going to guess that you've shared all your advice for others in a similar situation throughout this book. But here's your last chance. Do you have any other advice?

A: Go to physical therapy.

Acknowledgments

I've always thought the acknowledgement part of a book read a lot like the author's award acceptance speech. They thank this person or that and say the book wouldn't be possible without whomever they named. In truth, I never believed they meant what they wrote until I wrote my own book.

Now, I know that each acknowledgement is a heart-felt *thank you* to the individuals responsible for helping the author produce his or her best work.

Without the careful editing eye of Connie Anderson at WordsandDeedsInc.com, the focused proofreading of Ashley Patterson, and the formatting skills of Ann Aubitz at FuzionPrint; you literally would not be reading this book. These three women have worked so hard to ensure my diary-style ramblings come off as polished and complete thoughts, and the style and format of the book represent my vision. *Thank you.*

Also, if it weren't for my husband, you probably wouldn't be reading this. After a fifteen-year hiatus from writing, my husband encouraged me to start again. It's very likely that if I hadn't been in the habit of writing when I broke my neck, I wouldn't have journaled anything that happened and my whole experience would be forgotten. *Thank you.*

In terms of moral support, no one can top my parents. When I was a kid, my parents encouraged me to write and pursue my dreams. As an adult, they are my biggest cheerleaders and, when I'm injured, they are also my chauffeur and temporary care-givers to my kids. *Thank you.*

To my kids, thank you so much for almost always being angels. Your warm hugs, clever ideas, and naptime snuggles brighten my day. *Thank you.*

To my good friend and client, Alex, thank you so much for tackling the lofty job of writing a foreword to this book. It means so much to me that you would use your good name to give my book a little more credibility. *Thank you.*"

Finally, for all my friends and family members who have helped throughout this process, *thank you.* People who drove me, brought me food, lifted my spirits, listened to my rants, read through my book—I greatly appreciate everything you have done.

At the end of this whole process, I am left with one thought. I believe the Beatles (and Joe Cocker) said it best: "I get by with a little help from my friends."

Thank you so much, friends.

About the Author

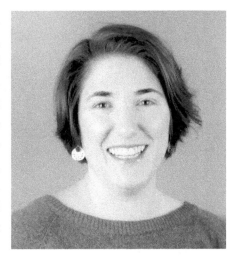

Sarah Stockett is a broken neck survivor, mom, wife, Pilates and yoga teacher, YouTuber, and blogger. When she's not teaching, she's researching the best ways to get rid of pain. To read more about yoga, Pilates, how to get rid of pain with exercise, and other tips to lead a happy, healthy life; visit her website: www.CustomPilatesandYoga.com.

CPSIA information can be obtained
at www.ICGtesting.com
Printed in the USA
LVHW040142100919
630431LV00007B/362

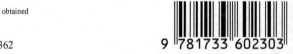